A House Called Helen

The development of hospice care for children

Second Edition

Jacqueline Worswick

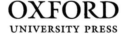

OXFORD
UNIVERSITY PRESS

*This book has been printed digitally and produced in a standard specification
in order to ensure its continuing availability*

OXFORD
UNIVERSITY PRESS

Great Clarendon Street, Oxford OX2 6DP

Oxford University Press is a department of the University of Oxford.
It furthers the University's objective of excellence in research, scholarship,
and education by publishing worldwide in

Oxford New York

Auckland   Cape Town Dar es Salaam   Hong Kong   Karachi
Kuala Lumpur Madrid Melbourne Mexico City   Nairobi
New Delhi Shanghai Taipei Toronto
With offices in
Argentina Austria Brazil Chile Czech Republic France Greece
Guatemala Hungary Italy Japan South Korea Poland Portugal
Singapore Switzerland Thailand Turkey Ukraine Vietnam

Oxford is a registered trade mark of Oxford University Press
in the UK and in certain other countries

Published in the United States
by Oxford University Press Inc., New York

ISBN   0-19-263235-3

Printed and bound by CPI Antony Rowe, Eastbourne

For Richard, who has lived through
everything I describe with me,
and without whose love, encouragement,
practical help and wise advice
I could never have completed this book;
for Catherine and Isobel, whose positive and
happy natures have sustained me throughout;
and for Helen, without whom this book,
like Helen House, would never have
come into being.

Contents

A *House Called Helen* documents a very important time in the history of hospice and palliative care services for children. It is an eloquent statement of the concerns and needs of families of children with chronic life-threatening and life-shortening illnesses. These have not changed since *A House Called Helen* was first written.

A House Called Helen challenges us to provide more effective services and approaches to the care of these children and their families. We cannot all build Helen Houses, (nor should we necessarily), but we can all take the philosophy that is manifest in the actions of everyone who works at Helen House and make it the cornerstone of care for children with chronic, life-threatening and life-shortening illnesses and their families.

The final chapter in this new edition provides a clear and thoughtful analysis of current issues in the developing field of paediatric palliative care, which should be read by all who have an interest in the field.

Myra Bluebond-Langner, Professor of Anthropology and Director of the Center for Children and Childhood Studies, Rutgers University, USA

Titles of books are always revealing. This one makes two statements, the first about a house or a home, and all that means in terms of care and compassion and friendship. Secondly it is about an individual, a person, with feelings, anxiety, concerns and needs. This book puts these two aspects together and tells the story of a challenge which was presented, and which was tackled and overcome. For the reader it identifies the lessons to be learned and shared with others.

Professor Sir Kenneth Calman, KCB, FRSE, Vice-Chancellor and Warden, University of Durham and former Chief Medical Officer

This book tells the story of the foundation in the 1980s in Oxford of the first hospice for children and its first ten years. . . . It provides a great insight into the problems of professionals and carers. . . . It is a book that everyone, not just health care professionals, should read, but it will be of particular interest to those working with severely or terminally ill children. . . It is a book to be read, re-read and thought about. . . It is particularly relevant in today's political and economic climate.

Child Health (Journal of the Association of British Paediatric Nurses)

A House Called Helen tells the story of the first specialist unit for palliative care for children in England. ... The description of how the house functions and how problems are dealt with make this book of special interest to health care professionals. . . As for its 'philosophy', you can begin to feel it only as you read the book: it seems to be quite the opposite of a philosophy, rather a concrete attitude of welcome from one day to the next, based on a belief that only families know what is good for them and Helen House is there to welcome them along with their ill child. A book that must be read.

European Journal of Palliative Care

Written to help those who have come to regard her daughter's name as a beacon and the hospice as a role model, [this book] will doubtless make Oxfordshire even more proud of what has been achieved over more than a decade.

The Oxford Times

A House Called Helen describes the developing and guiding philosophy of a children's hospice. In this edition it shows how this first venture has led to the growth of a children's hospice movement in the UK. It describes the problems faced by professionals and carers seeking to provide support to children suffering from life threatening illness, and to their families, and gives clear insight into the needs of these families. This book will be essential reading for individuals training in the field of palliative care and is important for any professional or lay person involved in the care of seriously ill children.

Professor Clifford C. Bailey, Consultant Paediatric Oncologist, United Leeds Teaching Hospitals Trust and Director of Research and Development, NHS Executive, Northern and Yorkshire

Introduction

Helen House, the first hospice for children in the UK, opened in Oxford in 1982. My purpose in writing this book in 1993 was to provide a full and comprehensive account of how Helen House came into being, what it does and how it operates.

The last decade of the twentieth century saw a rapid growth in the number of children's hospices and corresponding important developments in the field of what has become known as paediatric palliative care. What began with one modest venture in Oxford has developed into a powerful drive to establish the position of respite and terminal hospice care for children in the portfolio of service provision. Since the guiding principles behind hospice care for children stemmed from the philosophy which informed the foundation of Helen House, it is more important now than ever it was for that philosophy to be clearly understood.

It is for this reason that the main text of the original edition of *A House Called Helen* remains unchanged, since it charts the development of this philosophy from its conception to its realization. In the book I describe how Helen House arose from a special bond of friendship between Mother Frances Dominica and our daughter Helen, my husband Richard and myself. I record how the idea for Helen House emerged and how this idea was then translated into reality. The book contains a brief biography of Frances and information about those others whose important contributions enabled Helen House to develop in the way it did. It records the events surrounding the foundation of the hospice and describes in detail how the hospice operated during the first decade of its existence. The role and contribution of those who work at Helen House is described, as are the thoughts of some of the families who have used the hospice. In the final chapter of the original edition (Chapter 8) I touch on some of the difficulties encountered by families caring, often over a long period, for a child with a life-limiting illness, and the role and attitudes of the caring professions and indeed of the public at large.

The first two chapters of the book focus on our daughter Helen's sudden illness and the events which followed. If I have described these at some length, it is because what we experienced with and through Helen led directly to the birth of Helen House. To understand Helen House, it is helpful to know something of the events and experiences that pointed to the need for it, shaped the philosophy behind it and, indeed, informed the practical process of translating that philosophy into reality. Moreover, it is not just the broad brush strokes of Helen House that were determined by our experience with Helen; the small, but far from insignificant, details were influenced directly by what we encountered and felt when we were suddenly catapulted, with Helen, into new territory – the world of very ill children and those who care for them.

In this edition, published seven years after the original, I have added a new chapter, *Into the New Millennium*. This reviews the growth of children's hospices, reflects on their coming of age and the accompanying responsibilities and challenges, and considers some current and future issues in children's hospice care.

I should like to mark this new edition by expressing my appreciation to the many people who have written to me in the years since my book was first published. Moreover, preparing the final chapter has given me the opportunity to renew friendships and make new contacts with a wide range of people involved in children's palliative care. I am particularly grateful to the individuals who have given of their time so generously to talk to me and provide me with information, among them Helen Bennett, Bronwen Bennett, Izzy Bowles, Graham Collins, Jayne Dulson, David Featherstone, Margret Hartkopf, Lenore Hill, Kath Jones, Frances Kraus, Angela Mercer, Filomena Nalewajek, John Overton, Erika Richardson, Mandy Robbins, Meg Roberts and Dame Cicely Saunders.

Introduction

I should like to repeat my thanks to all the individuals mentioned in the original text who encouraged me at the outset in the writing of this book and provided me with information, in particular Sister Frances, Edith Anthem, Roger Burne and Michael Garside. I owe a particular debt of gratitude to Nigel Barklie for his photographs, to all the team at Helen House for their input and to the many families who talked to me with great warmth and openness.

Maturity and coming of age is a time for reflection, for taking stock, for considering what you wish to do with the time ahead. It may be that in this millennium children's hospices expand their role and enter new fields, developing 'hospice at home' services, for example, or providing education and training for other service providers. It may be that they increasingly adopt an advocacy role in relation to families, seeking to 'broker' comprehensive and tailor-made care arrangements, extending beyond what they themselves can offer, for children with life-limiting illnesses. Exactly how children's hospice care may develop is hard to predict. More important, though, than whether children's hospices focus exclusively on their core function or, alternatively, broaden their remit, is the approach and attitude which I hope will continue to inform what they do.

Helen House came into being in response to a clear and obvious need which it sought, quite simply, to address; the link between need and provision was close. This untrammelled and direct link is an essential feature of children's hospices. The challenge facing them as they enter their mature phase is how best to ensure that straightforwardness and simplicity are not clouded, that the wisdom and knowledge that come with maturity are yet accompanied by the refreshing directness, responsiveness and sharpness of vision so characteristic of childhood and early years.

Jacqueline Worswick
November 2000

1

Helen's Illness

'Other happy memories of that day are largely eclipsed by that unobliterable image of your little daughter's peaceful, happy and somehow wise-far-beyond-her-years face before the font . . . I think all of us at the christening party were knit together by our love for you and our admiration of your lovely little daughter. What will her gifts and talents be, I do wonder. Of her sweetness and reasonableness one is somehow already well apprised.' (From a letter from Belinda, Helen's Godmother, April 1976.)

At Helen's christening in Nottinghamshire her godparents and the friends and relations gathered to wish her well on her journey through life could hardly have guessed how short her active, well life was destined to be.

Helen was admitted to hospital in August 1978, barely two and a half years after that happy christening party. We were about to go on holiday to Cornwall and we were looking forward to relaxing; I was expecting our second child and had been feeling far from well, and Helen had shown mild symptoms of being under the weather, on and off, over several weeks. She had had sudden bouts of vomiting and had seemed rather tired and listless at times. She had also taken to crying at any loud noise and had fallen over a couple of times. We had taken her to the doctor several times and on one occasion, after a particularly spectacular fall down the stairs at her grandparents' house, we had taken her for an examination and X-rays at the hospital casualty department. On each occasion we had left, having been assured all was well. As our holiday approached, we felt we would all benefit from lazy hours on Cornish beaches.

A House Called Helen

However, the day before we were due to leave, Helen was suddenly very unwell; she was desperately pale and asked to 'go to her cot'. There she dozed fitfully, tossing about violently. When, in the afternoon, I found I could not rouse her easily, I rang our GP, who came immediately and, after examining Helen, wrote a letter referring us to the head injury specialist at the Radcliffe Infirmary casualty department. I had rung Richard at work and he had come home at once and in the late afternoon we set off, with Helen in my arms, for the hospital. Helen was never to return home able to play with the toys she left strewn around the sitting room or to stroke the cat who stared at us reproachfully as we hurried out that evening.

In the casualty department that evening we were fortunate to meet a young houseman who, when he examined Helen and looked closely into her eyes with an ophthalmoscope, felt that there were signs of severe pressure on the back of the eyes. He arranged for Helen to be admitted to hospital and for a brain scan to be done that evening.

At ten o'clock we received devastating news. I remember vividly that we were standing next to the illuminated goldfish tank in the children's ward when the houseman we had met in casualty came and told us that the scan had revealed that Helen had a very large tumour in the left ventricle of her brain. Ironically, the brightly coloured tropical fish, whose endless gentle circlings through clear water were meant to be both cheering and soothing to patients and visitors to the ward, were the helpless witnesses of a meeting which sent our normally cheerful spirits plummeting and threw our emotions into chaos. We were advised that Helen should have an emergency operation the next day to remove the tumour, although of course at that stage it was impossible to know whether the tumour was cancerous or benign. What was certain was that left where it was it would exert such pressure on the brain and do such damage as to kill Helen. We felt we had no option but to consent to the operation. I remember Richard asking the houseman who had had the unenviable task of breaking this news to us, 'Do children who have brain tumour operations like this usually recover?' The houseman answered, 'Some do, some don't.' Indefinite as this answer may seem, it was the most straightforward and unequivocal answer that we were to receive from any doctor over the next six awful months.

Helen was attached to a drip and tucked up in a cot in the children's ward. We said we would like to stay with her in hospital and, after some discussion, we were shown to a room in the nurses' wing where we could sleep. It was a long walk back along bleak corridors and up concrete stairs to reach Helen, and this underlined our separation from all we had previously known; at home Helen's bedroom was next to ours.

Somehow the night passed. In the morning we were told that Helen's operation was scheduled for twelve noon. She was obviously not allowed anything to eat or drink and she was amazingly patient and good as she watched other children tucking in to bowls of cereal. I promised her a cup of tea some time when her operation was over. (She has had that cup of tea many times, painstakingly slowly, from a spoon.) We stayed with her in turns all morning, each leaving her only to pick up belongings or to make telephone calls to friends and relatives to tell them the terrible news.

Because Helen was so calm and secure she was not given a pre-med injection. Instead, we carried her in our arms to the operating theatre and she was given the powerful injection that was to send her into deep unconsciousness while cradled in Richard's arms. As her eyes closed I remembered some anecdote that I had been meaning to tell her and I remember thinking: 'Oh dear, now Helen will never know about that.' At one level, therefore, I must have known that Helen would never again be well. How then we could subsequently have spent so many hours, days and weeks stimulating her and working to help her regain her faculties must strike many as very strange. There is no reason in these matters and hope is certainly unfettered by logic.

A House Called Helen

Helen's operation lasted four hours. We spent much of that time sitting on a grim metal balcony outside the children's ward, alone with our thoughts and fears, each looking to the other for reassurance. After four hours, we were told the operation was over and that Helen was in the recovery unit. Not long after that we were told that she was being moved to the special (intensive) care unit. We sat on stunted little wooden benches outside the special care unit, waiting to be told we could go in and see her. The young houseman who had admitted Helen to hospital and whom we regarded as our friend, simply, I think, because he had seen Helen conscious and talking before her operation, came and told us that we could now go in and see Helen but 'she was having a little trouble with her breathing'. I cannot describe how we felt at these words; breathing is such a basic and vital activity. We went into the special care unit. Helen lay on a snowy white bed, still in her own (green!) vest with her head swathed in bandages and wired up to numerous instruments we had never seen before but with which we were soon to become very familiar. On her face was a little oxygen mask. The doctors were not sure, they said, whether she could hear and understand what they were saying; perhaps we would like to try talking to Helen? We needed no directives. We took her little hands and told her to squeeze our fingers. She squeezed hard. Richard asked if she would like her teddy next to her. She firmly indicated that she would not. Then she suddenly put up one small hand, half pulled off her oxygen mask and spoke to us. Her words were not words of complaint, nor did she demand help or comfort. She said simply: 'I love you. I want music.' It was as though *she* were reassuring *us*. These were the last words she ever spoke. Her face began to twitch convulsively and she quickly lost consciousness. She was to remain in a coma for several months.

Helen spent the next ten days in the special care unit. During the night after her operation she very nearly died and for the first few days she was very ill indeed. The days she was in the special care unit were pervaded by a sense of timelessness; days and nights merged, with none of the landmarks which normally stake out a daily routine. The sense of timelessness was further heightened by the constant care Helen received, twenty-four hours non-stop; every barely perceptible change in her breathing or in her temperature was charted and observed. There was a special care nurse constantly at her side, day and night, alert to any movement or flicker.

Although Helen was clearly desperately ill, initially on a ventilator and with her temperature fluctuating violently, that period while she was in special care was in many ways easier to bear than the subsequent weeks on the ward. Special care, though it obviously suggested special need, implied that Helen was still the focus of great effort and medical attention. Backed up by all the technical wizardry, she might well recover. Our sense of shock was paralysing, but shock is a temporary state and one from which one emerges, and this suggested there was still hope.

Inevitably, for the hospital staff Helen was, during those days in the special care unit and later during the weeks on the ward, first and foremost a medical case. She was, after all, there because she had had a brain tumour, not because she was our Helen with her particular ways and characteristics. For this reason perhaps, we found the visits paid to Helen by the hospital chaplain reassuring; he spoke words from the Bible and prayer book over her inert and hot little body, words which in no way related to her as a medical case but which comforted us as parents of a child whose body might be impaired but whose person had a hold on our affections which went far deeper than that. Helen could not be cured by the words of Psalm 121 but the reading aloud of those words by the chaplain was an acknowledgment of all that Helen was, in herself and to us, irrespective of her medical condition.

It was when Helen had been in the special care unit for several days that I first met Frances, then Mother Frances Dominica, the Reverend Mother of All Saints Convent, an Anglican convent in East Oxford. Since so much has sprung from our meeting and the close friendship that developed between us, it is sobering to think how dependent on chance, and how fragile, were the links which brought us together. Two days after Helen's initial operation I had telephoned her godmother in London to tell her the terrible news about Helen. Belinda urged me to report back the next day. When I did, she told me that a friend of hers knew someone who knew someone in Oxford whom I might find it helpful to talk to. This person was called Mother Frances Dominica and her phone number was . . . I automatically wrote down the name and number on a scrap of paper and stuffed it in my pocket.

I told Richard about Belinda's message, and the next day said I was going to ring Mother Frances Dominica. Richard has often said since that he could not really see the point but he desperately wanted me to do anything that might bring me (and therefore him) any comfort or help. I rang. Frances was not there. I left a message saying I would ring again. How easily I might not have done; when you are in desperate circumstances and looking outwards for help, any seeming rejection from the direction you are looking in (even if the rejection is not intentional but results merely from a physical unavailability) is enough to make you give up. (That is why, incidentally, helplines, if they are to be sure of helping, must offer help non-stop.) The next day I left Richard at Helen's bedside, where Helen lay with eyes closed, hot and completely still and now without her one 'personalizing item' – her own vest – and went to ring Frances again. This time I spoke to her and in a very brief conversation we arranged that she would come and meet me the next day in the hospital foyer and we would go back to the convent for a while to talk.

Mother Frances Dominica: the combined maternal and religious overtones of the name conjured up in my mind a picture of a benign, spreading, cottage-loaf figure, radiating inner certainty. Fortunately Frances was wearing a black habit when I first met her at the hospital entrance; I might well not have recognized her otherwise. Her inner 'certainty' was translated into dynamism and energy; we walked briskly to her car where she introduced me to her dog and donned a stylish pair of sunglasses before steering her way nippily through the traffic and back to All Saints Convent. Over the next few weeks Richard and I had to adapt several stereotype pictures we held in our minds; that of the Reverend Mother was the first to go.

I shall never forget that afternoon I spent with Frances in the convent. I talked of Helen; I told Frances about our beloved only daughter, of her smile, her actions, her love of music, her funny little ways, the intense joy we felt in her company, her singing, her happiness. The pain of describing our vibrant Helen, while before me was the picture of her unconscious and still little body in the special care unit, was acute, yet brought with it real comfort. I realized fully how deeply shocking had been the sudden, brutal transformation, as much the result of environment as of circumstances, of Helen the person into Helen the medical case. To talk to somebody outside the hospital and also outside the immediate circle of relatives, someone who wanted to get an idea of what the real Helen was like, was hugely comforting. The comfort was the greater because from the start Frances and I felt a great affinity; I knew that, though tragedy had caused us to meet, a shared outlook would make us want to consolidate that meeting into friendship.

Some of the hardest experiences over the early weeks of Helen's illness were the visits we made back to our home in Abingdon. We were still living in the hospital so as to be near Helen night and day but obviously needed to go home on occasion to fetch clothes, do laundry and pick up post. Our first visit back to the house which had been the scene of all the 'active firsts' in Helen's life – her first words, first steps, first birthday party – and where all her toys and belongings lay as she had left them was acutely painful. The house was full of Helen's presence and character. Returning to it, albeit temporarily, also underlined that what had happened to Helen

19

was for real, not some aberration in an unreal clinical environment. What had happened to her had somehow to be fitted into our own world, or rather our own world had somehow got to be adjusted to include it. On that first visit we shut the front door behind us and wept uncontrollably; the physical pain of Helen's cruel removal from our familiar world was intense. We then picked a bunch of sweet peas for Helen from the garden, to vie with the clinical odours of the special care unit, and returned to the hospital.

When, after a little over a week, Helen was able to breathe without the aid of a ventilator and was taken off all life support machinery, it was suggested that, although she was still in the deep coma into which she had sunk shortly after the operation, she should be moved on to the ward. A decision was taken then which was to have unimagined consequences for us over the next few months; because Helen was so little the doctor arranged for her to be moved on to the children's medical ward, rather than on to a neurosurgical ward. He said, much later, that he had thought the environment of the busy children's ward would be more cheerful for us all.

We found Helen's move on to the children's ward very painful. It was as though Helen were being put out to pasture. While she had been in intensive care she had received what the title suggests. The intense activity and interest surrounding her had come some way towards matching the intensity of our feelings towards her and the intensity of any parent's belief that their child is special. From now on Helen would be, as we saw it, minded and kept comfortable (largely, as it later turned out, through our own efforts and ministrations) and would recover (or not) largely unaided. She remained a medical case, which in itself was painful to us, with the additional pain of her no longer even being a *special* medical case.

The ward Helen was moved to was a busy general children's ward in an old building. The staffing level at the best of times was barely adequate to cope with the demands of the wide variety of young patients and their families, all requiring very different treatment and approaches. For long-term patients and their families the fairly rapid turnover of nursing staff in particular, as student nurses came and went for relatively short training spells, was an added frustration. Another stereotype we held in our mind was soon toppled – that of the calm, competent, all-knowing nurse, bristling with starch and practical skills, who would take things in hand. While we of course wanted to be closely involved in Helen's care, the heavy reliance on us in all aspects of Helen's day-to-day care was both anxiety-inducing and physically exhausting. Of course it was understandable; we were there most of the time, we appeared competent; there were other children who urgently required attention and who were alone; what could be more logical than to leave us to get on with caring for Helen?

The routine of a crowded and understaffed ward in a busy hospital is inevitably geared up to coping with large numbers and, on occasion, with a sudden influx of patients. It cannot bow to individual preferences. This is obviously very 'depersonalizing'. In this context the staff have to make blanket decisions even in the non-medical areas. An example: we are dealing with children, many fairly advanced along the road to recovery; children need to be entertained; the most common, and easiest, source of entertainment in the land is television; therefore, during leisure hours, televisions should be switched on all around the ward. The noise level was incredible and we found ourselves longing for the quiet (albeit often a deeply sad one) of a neurosurgical ward. Later on, when we were able to spoon-feed Helen with liquidized food, the unyielding timetable of the meals trolley seemed bent on undermining all our desperate attempts to promote Helen's comfort and peace. If Helen had just fallen asleep after a relaxing session of physiotherapy or a bed bath, she could not be left to sleep if the meals trolley arrived; she (or we on her behalf) must respond to its clarion call – and very metallic and noisy it was too!

Being virtually permanent fixtures on the ward we got to know, if only superficially, a large number of other parents.

A House Called Helen

In that alien setting where our only *raison d'être*, or the only seemingly relevant thing about us, was that we were the parents of a sick child, it was natural that we were drawn into discussing Helen, her illness, her condition, the prognosis, etc., with other parents. Many of them desperately wanted to discuss their child and his or her difficulties with us. The emotional strain of becoming involved, albeit very willingly, in the often intolerable suffering of other parents was immense. Often there were other, non-medical, problems allied to, arising from, or even, in a few cases, causing, the medical condition which had resulted in the child being on the ward. While we felt at times very much caught up in a system, we had the dispiriting feeling that that system was only scraping the surface of many of the problems we came face to face with.

During the long weeks and months Helen lay in her bed on the ward, initially totally still and deeply unconscious, later less deeply unconscious and able to cry, we felt an engulfing sense of isolation. We thirsted after information about Helen's condition, about tumours generally, about the working of the brain, and, back to Helen again, about the outlook for our daughter. We felt a desperate need to know, to discuss Helen's condition with doctors, to receive information direct from the horse's mouth, not filtered down fifth hand (via nurses who knew nurses who had worked in neurosurgery). We received conflicting messages and information which merely exacerbated our feelings of loneliness and fear. Helen's situation revealed a very fundamental breakdown in communications within the hospital, more especially between different 'specialties'. Helen was a neurosurgical case and therefore under a neurosurgeon; however, she was a patient on a children's ward and therefore in the care of paediatricians. She neatly straddled two specialties. The paediatricians were around a lot of the time, involving themselves in the day-to-day care of sick children. The neurosurgeons were not around; they were either operating, taking clinics or visiting patients on their own (i.e. neurosurgical) wards or perhaps in special care postoperatively. We longed to talk to a neurosurgeon and requested this of the doctors and the sisters on the children's ward. Our messages did not get through, were not passed on or were imperfectly relayed. Finally, in desperation, we went home one day and rang Helen's neurosurgeon's secretary from outside the hospital and she happily gave us an appointment to see him!

A further complicating factor which added to our difficulties was that on the night Helen was admitted to hospital in August the consultant 'on take' in case of dire emergency was a professor based at the John Radcliffe Hospital, a couple of miles away; Helen, because she was admitted during his on-take hours was therefore technically his patient. All the bands around her wrists, the labels on her drugs, her notes, bore the professor's name. However, he seldom came down to the Radcliffe Infirmary and certainly never once met Helen. Yet, because she was technically his patient, the results of any tests done on her were sent off to him at the John Radcliffe and inevitably, even when they did not actually get mislaid (as happened on one occasion) they were not available for us to see for long anxious days after we might have hoped to glean something from them.

Ironically, the very poor communication network within the hospital was causing us unimagined distress at the very same time as the competent nurse figure we had expected to run into at every rubber swing door seemed to have been supplanted by clipboard-armed figures, hell-bent on liaison! We felt exhausted by our sapping grief, by our efforts to do as much as we possibly could to get Helen better and to enhance her comfort, by our desperate attempts to find out what was happening (and might happen), by our concern for other families on the ward, and by the noise and impersonality of Helen's surroundings.

All this time Helen remained in a coma. However, we were told by the neurosurgical registrar who, after we had begged to have a chance to talk to him and had even left notes stuck to Helen's metal bed-frame in case he should come when we had slipped out for a meal, did finally come and talk to us on the ward, and also by Helen's surgeon when we managed to meet him, that the neurosurgical view was that Helen would get better, that she would emerge from her coma and make a 'worthwhile' recovery. The tumour, analysed a few days after the operation, had proved to be benign and it had been removed. The scale of the operation had been such as to cause serious trauma and to send Helen into a coma, but the neurosurgeons were optimistic. I remember a very aristocratic-looking, grave-faced Egyptian neurosurgeon standing by Helen's bed one wintry evening and saying: 'Helen will get better.' Strangely, although this did not turn out to be the case, we remember that doctor with affection and warmth because he gave us hope.

The views of neurosurgeons relating to recovery and prognosis are constructed within a longer time perspective than those of paediatricians. There was no hope (and, I have to say, little comment) on offer from the paediatricians. We felt torn between opposing views, but, I suppose inevitably, we had to ally ourselves with the position of greater hope for Helen's sake and for our own. In fact Helen underwent two subsequent minor operations and the hope that surged up in us after the first of these, when she returned to the ward making a noise, after the silence and immobility of weeks, was intoxicating. It trickled away over subsequent days as it became clear that, although Helen was less deeply unconscious, there was no significant change in her condition.

The ward continued to hum with activity. I remember the day an entire class of schoolchildren was admitted following a leak of gas from a fume cupboard during a science lesson. Fortunately none of them was much the worse for the incident and after an afternoon of observation and checks, television viewing, magazine reading and general hilarity, they were allowed to leave. Other patients, too, came and went fairly rapidly, often having received treatment which had cured them completely of whatever problem they had been suffering from.

The stark contrast between the dramatic and speedy cures we frequently witnessed on the ward (and which, of course, we rejoiced to see) and Helen's unchanging, or barely changing, condition, was acutely painful and increased our sense of isolation. An acute children's ward is not the place to try to come to terms with long-term, grave illness.

All this time we devoted ourselves not only to promoting Helen's basic physical comfort (and we had an unceasing battle on that front, especially when on two occasions Helen succumbed to the 'ward bug' and got gastroenteritis) but also to stimulating her mind and senses, to relating to Helen the person, inside that poor, ill little body. We made tapes of familiar sounds from home – the cat purring, the kettle whistling, Richard playing the violin, the ducks on the millstream outside quacking, and played these to her, along with tapes of the church bells ringing at the church where her grandfather was vicar. We played music tapes to her and talked and read aloud to her endlessly, or simply sat and stroked her little limbs.

Frances, who had visited Helen for the first time shortly after she had been moved onto the children's ward, visited us and Helen regularly and we were soon bound not only by a shared love of Helen but also by a deepening friendship. There was no danger that Frances, if we spoke of Helen's spirit, would fear we were 'going under' from the strain; she understood our need to relate to Helen on a spiritual dimension. Though she had never known Helen as a well child, she had no difficulty in relating to Helen as a person. This proved very difficult for others, especially the younger staff, to do, because Helen did not do any of the things you normally relate to; she did not smile or communicate in any obvious way. In this context I remember the effect of our bringing in a colour photograph of Helen as a well, smiling two-year-old and sticking it to the metal bed-frame above her head. There was an immediate easing of the atmosphere around us and we felt that suddenly the nurses related to Helen and to her, in their eyes now only temporarily quenched, personality. One nurse started squeezing fresh oranges to make Helen drinks with 'lots of vitamins in – they'll do her good'. Another made her a dress. I must emphasize here that there was a lot of kindness and warmth around us, though some of the most sustaining warmth and help came not from those with most experience and medical qualifications but from those who followed their own instincts of humanity and empathy.

For the medical staff in that hospital where Helen spent six long months and for doctors in general, I am sure, there are many strains and problems. Sitting for hours on end by Helen's bedside in a busy medical ward we had much time to reflect on the role of doctors and what we expect of them. Ask a child to tell you what a doctor is or does; he or she will probably tell you, in some way or another, that a doctor is someone who makes you better when you are poorly. If at any time you benefit from something, that something is often described as being 'just what the doctor ordered'. Doctors could be excused for believing that their patients and their patients' families judge and value them purely on the basis of their success in 'curing' their patients, in making them better.

From this belief, perhaps, springs the embarrassment some doctors display when a patient does not get better, and their inability to cope with this. Also, in a profession not, perhaps, noted for humility, there is possibly a reluctance to associate yourself with failure and a patient who does not get better often denotes failure to doctors, regardless of the skill, expertise, energy or (very important to patients this one!) humanity with which the doctor has treated the patient. This embarrassment on the part of medical staff, this understandable desire to be on the winning side and the inability to cope with patients not getting better, perhaps explains some of the things we suffered during Helen's hospital stay. The doctors on the ward did not come forward to talk about Helen. Interestingly, one of them wrote to us out of the blue several years later when Helen House opened and expressed, among other things, his regret that the doctors on the ward had left us alone as they did. 'We didn't know what to say to you', he wrote. (Amy, who cleaned the ward and who sang spirituals *fortissimo* in the broom cupboard, did not have the same problem.) The regular ward rounds usually by-passed Helen's bed. Such things inevitably added to our feeling of isolation.

Of course, in a busy ward where there are patients who can respond, who clearly can get better, it makes sense, if you are short of time and energy, to devote what time and energy you do have to those patients. We understood that, but could have wished that the more holistic approach, which we believe is now creeping into hospitals, had taken root before our beloved Helen was a patient in hospital.

We struggled day after day to salvage Helen's individuality and to preserve our feeling of being a real family with roots outside the hospital confines, in the world of emotions, ideas and day-to-day events. On a purely practical level things became increasingly difficult as the weeks passed. For the first couple of weeks of Helen's time in hospital Richard had been on annual leave (we had, after all, been supposed to be holidaying in Cornwall then) but after that he had had to return to work. We had moved back home and had attempted to pick up the threads of our, until then very happy, existence in Abingdon. Our second child, due in a couple of months, was very active inside me and I often felt exhausted.

We developed a sort of routine; Richard would often get up early and drive into the hospital in Oxford to wash, dress and feed Helen before turning round to go in the opposite direction to work. I would go in by bus every day to the hospital, getting there in the first half of the morning and leaving mid to late afternoon. After supper at home together, one or other of us would almost invariably return to the hospital to be with Helen until she was asleep and to sit and watch her sleeping and stroke her limbs. Looking back I realize it was an exhausting routine, but we would not have been happy with anything less. We were not, of course, happy with the routine we were following. Happiness was not, at that stage, something we knew; aching and quite exhausting grief, coupled with a strange determination and indefatigable perseverance and tenacity in everything relating to Helen, were our staple diet then. We felt, quite simply, utterly bereft.

Sometimes as we sat at Helen's bedside in those very bleak surroundings we would be overwhelmed by the awfulness of Helen's plight and by our unbearable pain. We were exhausted too from the violent see-sawing between hope and despair. We would start to weep. We quickly realized that our grief was quite simply considered out of place, that it needed to be hidden. What we came to call 'the Noddy screens' (very depressing, faded yellow screens with pictures of a grotesquely cheerful Noddy splashed all over them) were quickly pulled around Helen's bed and us. Our grief, discreet and quiet though it was, was clearly a threat to the social order, not a normal emotional response to a very tragic situation. Perhaps this is why on one or two such occasions when we had been tearful, the hospital social worker was wheeled in to ask us the unfailing question: 'How are things?' I realize it is a rare person indeed who can accept simply to be alongside you where you are emotionally, without being prescriptive as to where you should be, particularly in the hard-pressed situation of a busy hospital ward, but that is what we, and I am sure others on that ward, desperately needed.

Our second child was due at the end of November. When, two weeks after she was due, she still had not arrived, I was taken into the John Radcliffe Hospital to have the baby induced. Catherine arrived in the evening of a chill December day and we were flooded with love for her. At the same time, the intensity of our joy at her birth accentuated the rawness of our grief at what had happened to our first daughter, born almost exactly three years before. After spending a couple of hours with Catherine and me, Richard set off for the Radcliffe Infirmary to go and tell Helen, unconscious as she was, that she had a little sister. For the next ten days Richard spent his 'free' time commuting between two hospitals, catapulted from the joy and beaming faces of the maternity wards to the sadness and drawn expressions of the children's medical ward.

Five days after Catherine's birth Richard drove me down to the Radcliffe Infirmary to be with Helen on her third birthday. He had bought a chocolate cake and decorated it with candles and Helen's name in silver foil letters; we thought the light of the candles reflected off the foil might somehow reach her. I have a photograph of us all with a few relations and friends on that day. Helen had been lovingly dressed by a nurse in the sort of party dress you expect to see frothing up around a little girl as she falls, laughing, to the floor in a game of musical bumps. In the photograph, Helen, desperately pale and her body rigid, lies in Richard's arms. That afternoon we carried her down to the hospital chapel to attend the hospital carol service. As we sang carols and listened to Helen's surgeon reading the Christmas story we remembered the other lonely visits we had paid to that chapel in the days after Helen's operation. The suffering we carried into that chapel was, I suppose, some kind of prayer.

We were determined that we would all be together in our own home on Christmas Day and we put up and decorated a beautiful Christmas tree for our two little daughters. The hospital staff were happy to allow Helen to come home with us for a visit and it was agreed that she would spend a couple of days with us in Abingdon. When we carried her home, her little body was very stiff and in a sort of rigid spasm, as it was most of the time at that stage, and totally unyielding to stroking and gentle attempts to bend and relax the limbs. We struggled to generate joy, to shed an atmosphere of light and happiness over our little family group. We held both Helen and Catherine up to the Christmas tree to see the brightly coloured balls and lights and filled the room with beautiful Christmas music. Sadly, Helen was very distressed during the night and it was clear to us that she was in some additional pain and on Boxing Day morning we had to rush back to hospital with her.

A House Called Helen

Soon after that Christmas the weather turned bitterly cold and there was snow and ice on the roads. It was difficult to maintain our routine with Helen but we managed somehow. I would set off in the bright, frosty mornings with Catherine in a carrycot and spend several hours at Helen's bedside while Catherine slept in Sister's office. Fortunately Catherine was a very sunny and contented baby who quite simply never cried. Richard would spend long, sad evenings at Helen's bedside.

In the first weeks of her life Catherine was inundated with presents and more people than we thought we knew wrote to us expressing their delight at her birth. They were, of course, delighted at her birth, but sending us such loving and congratulatory messages was also for them a way of telling us how desperately sad they were at what had happened to Helen. We appreciated all this love but also felt desperately protective of Helen and her need, and ours, for love to be poured directly onto her. 'At last we have something we can rejoice with you over'; one of the many messages we received, this seemed to suggest that from now on Catherine's health, happiness and fitness would be a useful distraction from the tragedy that was Helen. (Helen House was later to be used in the same way.) We did feel that in some people's eyes we should be at home with Catherine all the time, being positive, instead of being 'morbid' and hanging around the hospital! Of course, Catherine had a right to our undivided love and attention at times – and she frequently got it in rich measure – but we still had two daughters and we loved them both equally. We often felt drained by the very conflicting emotions those two little creatures and their contrasting conditions aroused in us and this was all the more poignant because these emotions were there all the time, raging within us simultaneously.

Frances continued to offer us immense support. She visited us at home and sometimes would go in to visit Helen and give her her supper to relieve us. It was very important to us, if for some reason we simply could not get to Helen's bedside, to know that someone who really loved Helen, who entered into our worries and hopes on her behalf and who knew little things like what song Helen liked to have sung to her as she fell asleep (and was prepared to sing it!) was with her. We talked to Frances about the sliver of fear that I know had always been there but which was becoming more insistent in its stabbings at our consciousness – the fear that Helen would not get better.

Towards the end of January, following a talk we had with Helen's neurosurgeon, it was agreed that it would be useful to do a brain scan on Helen. It should by now be possible to discover quite a lot from such a scan. The neurosurgeon explained that until that point a scan would not have been very useful or revealing; brain tissue does not show up as damaged until some time after the damage has been done. The shrinkage of the tissue, which is indicative of damage, is not immediately apparent. We felt both apprehensive and hugely relieved at the thought that we would perhaps soon know something definite about Helen's condition and have some real indication of the outlook for her. Of course we longed to have our wildest hopes consolidated but we also longed to have them quenched if there were nothing to sustain them. In the limbo we seemed to be living in we simply did not know how to direct our energies to Helen's greatest benefit.

Helen duly had a brain scan. The suspense surrounding the results was made all the more agonizing because the test results were, in accordance with the bureaucracy of the organization, sent off unseen by anyone in the hospital where Helen was and where we lurched from hope to despair, to the hospital where 'her' doctor (i.e. the one on take on the fateful night she was admitted to hospital) was based. The results were furthermore 'temporarily mislaid in transit'. Each day we thought we would at last know what Helen's chances of recovery were; each day, for more than a week, these hopes were dashed. Finally it was arranged that we would go to see Helen's surgeon on the following Saturday morning to discuss the scan findings with him.

A House Called Helen

As we walked into his office I knew at once that from then on it really was just Helen and us; looking at the surgeon's face I knew he had no hope to offer us. As he swallowed twice during the sentence in which he told us that the outlook for Helen was 'very bleak' and that she was 'unlikely to live for very long', I felt desperately sorry for him and longed to reassure him and tell him that we really were all right and that we would cope. I liked him because in offering us no hope he was clearly deeply affected by the enormity of what he was saying.

The moment we knew that there was nothing more that could be done medically in hospital to make Helen get better we knew that she should be at home with us. She belonged within the warmth and love of her own family. In a strange way there was, even within the pain and shock of the news we had received only moments before, a sense of relief that at last we knew where to concentrate our best efforts, that the needs of Helen the person would once again clearly override the problems of Helen the medical case.

We returned to the ward, where we briefly told the nurse in charge the basic findings of the scan. We asked if we could take Helen home for the weekend and if we could have the necessary drugs for her. (She needed muscle relaxants and drugs for epilepsy; since the operation she had suffered epileptic fits.) I think the nurse must have guessed our intention. She suggested we took enough drugs for a week 'to be on the safe side'. We bundled Helen up in a blanket and carried her downstairs and out into the crisp February air and into our car. She never again returned to hospital.

Our carrying her lovingly away with us and home like that was prompted by two instinctive feelings. We were very conscious of one of these; we were less consciously aware of the other but in retrospect we realize its instinctive prompting was very sound. First, Helen was our dearly beloved daughter and she should be at home with us. The increased hopelessness of her situation made her need of our love and care all the greater. Second, if we had waited for meetings to be set up between social workers, health visitors, psychologists and other 'experts', to discuss what should be done about 'the Helen situation' and whether 'the parents' could cope with her at home, the 'paper evidence' – the discussion based on case lore, questionable statistics and research – might well have stifled the 'human evidence' – that we loved Helen dearly, we needed her, she needed us and that yes, it would be very hard to look after her at home, but we would do it.

Almost six months to the day after the sunny August day when we had driven her to hospital, we drove Helen back home. Much had changed but not our deep love for her.

2

Home from Hospital

When we closed our own front door behind us on the morning we brought Helen home from hospital for good we felt an enormous sense of relief. For the first time for weeks and months our confidence in the rightness of what we were doing for our daughter was untempered by any need to seek confirmation from an expert. We felt, for the first time in ages, truly on home ground. At the same time we felt hugely vulnerable. The contrast between the hospital and our home was, while comforting in one sense, daunting in another. In hospital, although we did much of the practical day-to-day caring for Helen ourselves, there was the feeling that there existed a 'safety net', a backup system of machinery and medical expertise on tap should anything go wrong; our home was full of love and reassuringly familiar sounds and smells and our efforts to make Helen comfortable would, we knew, be unremitting, but our house lacked any medical facilities and support. We were suddenly on our own and although this choice had been ours, our shock at the reality was immense.

Moreover, simply being at home all the time reminded us forcefully of our other responsibilities, duties and concerns. We felt suddenly very busy and tired. On a purely practical level, the house we lived in then presented us with some difficult problems. We had moved into it with Helen as a baby just over two years previously when it had, to employ the language of coy understatement dear to estate agents, 'offered considerable scope for imaginative and sympathetic modernization'. We had already undertaken some major repairs and adaptations, some only recently completed, but there was still much to be done. Carrying out major building work on your house and garden and caring for a very ill child at home at the same time is not to be recommended, but this was to be an experience we had to face on a couple of occasions over the next few years. However, some aspects of the basic design, layout and situation of our much-loved house and garden simply could not be adapted to suit our changed needs. Precipitous, narrow, winding wooden stairs was one charming but impractical feature of our lovely old house. A front door, with two steep steps, opening directly onto the street, was another. No guaranteed parking near the house made taking Helen out very difficult. A very small bathroom with little room to manoeuvre was suddenly very impractical.

Helen's condition when we brought her home from hospital gave the idiom 'a bundle of nerves' real meaning. It was as though her little body was made up entirely of nerves, every one of which was exposed and suffered from any physical contact or movement. She was very distressed; picking her up sent her into rigid spasms and set her crying noisily; putting her down often provoked the startle reflex seen with new-born babies who, when put down suddenly, throw their arms back. She found loud and harsh noises very distressing; the telephone ringing or saucepans clashing set her crying. (In hospital, the metal cot sides being briskly lowered had caused her huge distress.) Her stiff, tense little body made changing and washing her very difficult. Although she was no longer tube-fed, feeding her was not a relaxed and happy experience. All Helen's food had to be liquidized and because she had such trouble swallowing we felt feeding her was more like an invasion than the comforting, bonding experience it is with the small babies whom, in her helplessness, Helen now so closely resembled. Because giving her fluids was so difficult, but so vital, we experimented with jelly, hoping its semi-solid state would be easier for her to cope with than liquids.

Giving her her drugs three times a day was an ordeal. Presumably because she was a child, she had been prescribed her medicines in syrup form and the memory of struggling to pour largish quantities of two different thick, sickly medicines, reminiscent in smell of nail varnish, down little Helen's throat, haunts us both. She choked and coughed however slowly and tenderly we tried to carry out the procedure. Later, when it occurred to us to ask if we could have her drugs in tablet form, things were easier (though never simple) and there was the added bonus of not fearing that the medicines were rotting Helen's teeth and damaging her gums.

As well as being unbelievably edgy, tense and easily distressed, Helen was also at that stage very weak. We brought her cot bed into our bedroom and she slept next to our bed for several months so that we could check on her frequently and be alert to any changes in her breathing and also be with her immediately if she had an epileptic fit. The boundaries between day and night were not clearly staked out for little Helen; she spent her days lying down and often dozing and all that distinguished night from day was a change of garments and a change of lying place, relative silence and, perhaps, some sense of a difference in light. Though it was hard to be sure about this, her vision (which we attempted to stimulate with mirrors, candles, lights and bright objects) probably encompassed a difference between light and darkness. How we yearned for the clear leap from night to day, heralded in the past by Helen's happy singing in her cot as she greeted a new day. Catherine very kindly assumed the mantle and provided us with astonishing morning concerts which exhausted her to such a degree that she then conveniently fell asleep again, giving us time to wash and dress Helen, but that was later.

Our feeling of vulnerability and isolation was increased by the fact that, because Helen was at first so noisy and distressed, it was almost impossible to have relaxed conversations with friends, either in person or on the telephone. Our GP visited us, often spontaneously, and from him we received not only medical advice and help but also sympathy and friendship, for which we were then, and remain today, very grateful. One thread of continuity with the recent past and with Helen's hospital stay was provided by the community paediatric physiotherapist who called regularly, once a week, to work on Helen's trunk and limbs. She had visited Helen in hospital to get to know her and assess her needs and soon after Helen came home she began coming to see her there. Her visits were very welcome; not only did we feel her active therapy was benefiting Helen greatly and enhancing her comfort, but we found her concern, interest and empathy and her very obvious and growing love for Helen very sustaining. On her first visit to our house she was overcome by seeing Helen in her own home and started weeping. Paradoxically, this brought us more comfort than anything had done for weeks. By entering into what we felt about Helen and acknowledging the awfulness of Helen's (and our) situation, Bronwen made us feel supported and less like alien beings in a world where one's primary duty was to be cheerful.

Richard found returning to work, which he did three weeks after Helen was first taken ill, very difficult. Many parents will have experienced that sense of strangeness, of disorientation you get when you first emerge into the wide world again after the birth of a baby. It seems quite simply astonishing that, given the amazing and wonderful event that has just occurred in your personal world, the world outside can be carrying on as though nothing had changed. Richard, his family life thrown into confusion by what had happened to Helen, full of grief and exhausted as we swung backwards and forwards between hope and fear, had to return to work and try to believe in the unchanged importance and significance of the tasks before him. It was very hard for him, all the more so as he did somehow manage to put on a brave face. He remembers a colleague remarking to him one day, 'You certainly seem to have got over things very well.' Similarly, at a later stage, because, I suppose, I was out and about and doing ordinary things like shopping, it was assumed I had put Helen's tragedy behind me. 'You've managed to take it in your stride', was what was said to me one day in Abingdon shopping precinct – and this was a statement, not a tentative question! Could anybody take a tragedy like Helen's in their stride?

Related to this was the astonishing readiness of some people to imagine that the birth of Catherine had somehow compensated fully for the illness and helplessness of Helen. Friends whose son died of cancer and who had a daughter a couple of months later comment on how extraordinary it is that some people clearly feel that the arrival of a new baby can fill the hole left by the death of another child. No child can ever be replaced; the pain you suffer for one cannot be neatly cancelled out by the joy you find in another.

Apart from the greatly appreciated visits of the physiotherapist, we were offered very little practical help and support in the home, though much later, after the birth of our third daughter, a nurse called once a week to help me bath Helen. This is not to say we did not receive visits from professionals who might have provided some assistance with what were, to us, bewilderingly new concerns but which we naively assumed they knew about and indeed welfare services provided for. One of the first visits we received was from an occupational therapist who was accompanied by a young trainee. After a long and friendly discussion over a cup of coffee we concluded that there was probably very little that could be supplied at that stage to help us look after Helen. However, we said we had some difficulty in bathing her and Richard asked whether there might be some sort of bath aid or headrest that we could use to provide some support when we washed her. He made a sketch of the kind of thing that might help. Our visitors eagerly measured the dimensions of our bath and left, clutching Richard's sketch.

For weeks nothing happened. Six months later a man appeared at our door carrying a peculiar object; it was a broomstick with a rubber cap at each end. A large piece of foam rubber was attached half way down the stick. The man said apologetically that we would have to saw the stick to fit it in the bath and handed us a spare piece of foam rubber which he thought might be useful. Could this really be a bath aid provided by trained therapists? It was clear that the stick would be of no use but Richard felt that we should try out the spare piece of foam rubber. It offered no firm support for Helen's head; moreover, it absorbed the bath water like a sponge and was impossible to dry. The following day it had developed an unpleasant smell. A few days later we returned the device, together with two ramps which had been delivered by registered post and were supposed to help get Helen's wheelchair up the steps to the front door but which did not fit. Despite its comic overtones, this episode was a distressing waste of time, both ours and that of the welfare services.

Another incident which also proved to be unproductive was a visit to our house by a community physician who arranged to see us to discuss arrangements for Helen at home. Richard talked to her while I was looking after Helen and Catherine in another room. It was rapidly apparent that she knew very little about Helen's illness and the background to it. She started by asking questions about Helen's birth and then homed in on the relationship between Richard and me. Richard was mildly astonished by the drift of the conversation; he could see little point in discussing the intimacies of our marriage in this context (and indeed had no wish to do so!) He asked what practical help might be available to us. In particular he explained that we were anxious about who might look after Helen if either of us were taken ill or if we wanted to have a break with Catherine. The community physician recommended that Helen should stay in a hospital called Bradwell Grove although, to our astonishment, she said that she herself had never visited it. She was unable to offer any suggestions for help with nursing at home or any other type of support. Richard made a note of the name of the hospital and the community physician left without seeing Helen.

We have always tried to keep an open mind and avoid dismissing things out of hand and, indeed, have tried to explore any avenues which might lead to improvements in, or simply an easing of, the inevitable problems surrounding our life with Helen. So it was that we determined to visit Bradwell Grove, the hospital recommended, though never visited, by the community physician. Our arranged visit took place on a blustery day of scudding clouds. Bradwell Grove turned out to be a ramshackle complex of single-storey huts, built during the Second World War. At the time of our visit it housed a long-term mental hospital for adults with, in addition, one children's ward. The decrepit, tatty and insubstantial appearance of the temporary buildings belied the substantial and very long-term problems of the sad individuals to whom they were 'home'. Our hearts sank as we parked the car and went in.

We were shown into an office where we met a doctor, a child psychiatrist based at the Park Hospital who called regularly at Bradwell Grove to offer advice and guidance on the care of children in the children's ward. We told her about Helen, how we cared for her at home, and how we had been advised to consider Bradwell Grove as a possible place for respite care for her. She introduced us to a nurse who worked on the children's ward and asked him to show us round. As we walked along the long draughty passages to the children's ward we passed several mentally handicapped adults aimlessly wandering the corridors. They were clearly very excited by our presence; the excitement of a visitor was obviously a highlight in an existence usually starved of incident.

We found our visit to the children's ward unbearably sad. Great effort had clearly gone into the room's decoration; it had been made to look cheerful and bright colours had been used in an attempt to mask the dreary dilapidation of the flimsy buildings. Some of the children on the ward were permanently resident there; others came to stay for short periods. Of the permanent residents, some had been rejected by their parents and families and never received a visit. Several were totally helpless and we shall never forget one boy, blind and deaf and contorted into a ball, who lay wrapped in his own dark, silent world, seemingly beyond the reach of such care and affection as he might receive.

The staff nurse described some of the difficulties he and his staff faced (without, I may say, even a hint of complaint or self-pity) and touched on ethical questions such as their struggles to keep children alive *in loco parentis*. He spoke of his charges with great gentleness and concern and we were impressed by his positive spirit, his dedication and by the efforts of the staff in general. However, nothing could dispel our deep sadness, the overriding feeling that we were in a twilight world, where unfortunate individuals clung to the fringes of life, largely forgotten by those in the mainstream.

We thanked those who had welcomed us and shown us round, told them we would think about what we had seen (it was something we would never be able to stop thinking about) and that we would be in touch. On our way home we stopped the car on the edge of a field, overlooking a broad sweep of countryside where birds wheeled in the air with poignant ease, and wept.

Later, we wrote to the doctor we had met at Bradwell Grove (who later was to play a part at Helen House) and thanked her for seeing us. We told her we did not feel that Bradwell Grove was quite what we were looking for for Helen. How useful understatement can be in times of pain.

Some weeks later I took Catherine to our GP's surgery with some minor ailment. I told our doctor that we had thought about respite care and that we had visited Bradwell Grove. We now felt we could not leave Helen and go away on holiday. He asked me whether it was the idea of leaving Helen at all that made us unable to go on holiday or if it was Bradwell Grove in particular that was the stumbling block. I told him it was the latter. He then told me that in that case we might like to consider an offer from his wife to look after Helen for a fortnight while we took Catherine on holiday. I was overcome. We had known our GP Richard and his wife Maureen a little in a non-professional capacity for some time (we had mutual friends and had met socially) but I felt quite simply stunned by Maureen's great kindness in offering to have Helen to stay. We accepted the offer and, almost a year after Helen was so suddenly taken ill, we took her baby sister Catherine for the seaside holiday Helen herself should have had the previous year. Maureen and Richard have continued to have Helen to stay each summer since then, thus enabling us to go away on a summer holiday with our other two daughters. Theirs is the sort of immense kindness and support whose special worth lies in its being unflaunted and straightforward. The only problem for us (if 'problem' is the right word in this context) is that the very matter-of-fact way they approach caring for Helen makes it seem so easy that we wonder if we make heavy weather of it!

In the early days of caring for Helen at home there was one problem which took up an inordinate amount of time and caused us much anxiety which we could well have done without. This related to the provision of a wheelchair for Helen. Towards the end of her period in hospital, when she had emerged from her initial deep coma, Helen became able to take liquidized food from a spoon. In order for this difficult feeding operation to be carried out she needed to be held sufficiently upright not to choke. However, as she was unable any longer to support her neck and body, she could not sit in any normal type of chair. One day the hospital physiotherapist, who had been regularly and devotedly attending Helen, happened to go to a demonstration of equipment for the disabled and she identified a small wheelchair which she felt would provide Helen with sufficient support for her to sit in a slightly reclined position. The wheelchair was duly prescribed for her by her consultant neurosurgeon.

Several weeks later, when at last we were at home with Helen, we were in desperate need of a chair to support her. Richard made enquiries and found that, for some inexplicable reason, the wheelchair had not actually been ordered as intended. We were relieved when the physiotherapist who had originally identified the chair arranged with the firm who supplied it to lend us one 'on approval' until the paperwork for the order from the hospital had been processed.

However, it soon proved not to be as simple as this. After many telephone calls to the hospital, the Artificial Limb and Appliances Centre (ALAC) and DHSS offices in Oxford, Preston and Blackpool, we discovered that, although the chair had been prescribed, it had not actually been ordered because, being a newly available chair, it was not on the 'approved list' of NHS chairs. The doctor at ALAC, who assured us that he would sort the matter out and that we should retain the chair that we had been lent on approval, subsequently informed us 'with regret' that we would have to pay for it.

Over the next few months we became embroiled in a battle with the DHSS which we fought for Helen but also as a matter of principle. We discovered that the DHSS had a 'wheelchair policy' and that under this policy children as disabled as Helen had the right to be provided with a wheelchair. Although no one disputed that the wheelchair prescribed for Helen was the only one which was remotely suitable for her, the DHSS refused to supply it. The reasons we were given shifted. It was not a 'standard' chair, yet it was agreed that no standard chair was suitable for Helen. It was an expensive chair, yet it was accepted that to adapt any other chair would be more expensive. Later on it was suggested that it might not be stable, yet Helen was totally paralysed and could not move on her own. While a highly active child might possibly have been able to tip the chair, this was not relevant in Helen's case. The same letter which warned us of the possible instability of the chair suggested we should apply to charitable foundations for financial assistance to buy it – strange advice if the chair was really thought to be unsafe!

We were sent the bill and we sent it back. The growing file of correspondence was sent backwards and forwards between Oxford and 'headquarters' in Blackpool. The dreadful letters we received were from people who had never seen Helen. All those who had and who were able therefore to assess her needs were adamant that the chair now in our possession was the only one remotely suitable for her.

Finally, six months later, we received a rather ungracious letter from 'headquarters' which said that 'after reconsidering all the circumstances' it had been agreed to supply Helen with the chair that had been prescribed for her. It was stressed that 'the decision was exceptional'. On top of the other things with which we were having to contend, we found the whole episode very distressing. We had never been on the receiving end of the social services before and we were upset by what appeared to us to be a total lack of common sense, humanity or flexibility. We had won in this case, as we were later to win in other battles for adequate provision for Helen, because we were articulate and we had persisted. However, the treatment we received was far from what we had imagined was provided by 'the welfare services'.

A friend who has a mentally handicapped son now in his mid-twenties who lives with her at home recently remarked, 'There are plenty of people who will come and see you and talk but no one who will actually do anything'. I am sure she, as we do, recognizes the importance of needs being properly assessed and information being gathered, but of course gathering information, while it perhaps shows recognition of a problem, does nothing in itself to solve that problem. To be of practical benefit, information must be acted upon appropriately. If it is not, the invasion of privacy the gathering entails is inexcusable. 'I can't help you if you won't tell me what's wrong' is a valid comment, but surely implicit in the comment is 'and when you've told me, I will help you'?

Ironically, in our experience it is often those same people, who will talk to you about your needs and then go away and provide nothing, who are most assured in their exhortations to you to make sure that you get out and about and carry on with life. There are clearly major resource problems in the provision of support services but there are fundamental flaws in the approach to such provision. An additional problem is that if you are impatient of the numerous fruitless interviews, often simply because you have your hands full with the problems of caring, you are deemed to be aloof and unco-operative.

While Helen was still in hospital we had, as I have mentioned, spent hours reading to her, talking to her, stimulating her through speech, sound, light and touch and doing things which we hoped would be beneficial to her and, indeed, perhaps give her some pleasure. A teacher friend who had known Helen ever since she was born and whom we had talked to about all this told us of someone she knew, a strong, capable, very positive and nice nursery nurse who was seeking some part-time work. Perhaps this person might help us in some way with caring for Helen and doing things with her on her return from hospital whenever that took place? We invited Hilary to our house and she went to see Helen in hospital. When we brought Helen home, Hilary was ready to help us.

We employed Hilary on a professional basis (although she soon became a good friend) and she came to our house on two mornings a week, for two hours at a time, to look after Helen but, more importantly (for us as well as for Helen, I readily acknowledge) to *do* things with her. There was no end to Hilary's positive energy and enthusiasm. As well as working with music and rhythm with Helen, she did a lot of sensory work with her and engaged her in finger and foot painting. She also cuddled her and learnt how to feed her and give her drinks. I felt reassured that there was now one other person apart from ourselves and Frances who was able to feed Helen and give her her drugs; we continued to feel vulnerable and sometimes wondered what would happen if we were suddenly both ill. We did often feel that, to quote Oscar Wilde's Lady Bracknell, 'health was our primary duty'! While Hilary was at home with Helen I could go out with Catherine, take her to the swings or to feed the ducks or do some shopping. Thus the only practical help we received, apart from the visits of the physiotherapist, had come through our own friends and our own initiatives. We feel for those who are less fortunate and who have to look to the caring professions for practical support.

Those first weeks, months, and indeed years at home with Helen and her lovely little sister, Catherine, were by no means given over entirely to sadness. It is amazing to me, looking back, to consider how much was happening in our lives at that period and how, too, we were propelled by what I suppose was a very basic, instinctive tendency towards happiness. That is not to say that we did not from time to time just crumple under our grief, sometimes at moments of particular strain, but often totally unexpectedly. We often felt bereft. Yet there was much that brought us great joy. Catherine was a source of indescribable pleasure; her sunny disposition, confidence and unquenchable delight in life, while a rather poignant reminder of her elder sister's early years, brought us great happiness. We enjoyed the company and kindness of many good friends. Richard had taken on new responsibilities at work which he found very stimulating and interesting and which meant he was visiting the EC headquarters in Brussels once a month for a few days. Life definitely went on – as we are always told it must.

There was a change in Helen over the first few months she was at home, which we felt was very significant on the human/emotional scale on which we considered her 'progress'. She gradually began to relax, to become less stiff, tense and edgy. It was as though, as I told Frances, she were thawing out in the warmth of the love by which she was surrounded in the security of her own home. At the same time she ceased to be distressed and noisy; picking her up and moving her no longer triggered crying but on the contrary became the almost certain way of comforting her and silencing the strange, plaintive crying noise she occasionally made when she was slightly uncomfortable or simply, we concluded, lonely. Her normal (i.e. usual) state became one of calm, even at times, we felt, of serenity. If we had sought any confirmation of the wisdom of bringing her home, this change alone would have provided it. We had been told very clearly that any 'real improvement' in Helen's condition was impossible, by which was meant improvement in her medical condition, progress towards cure, but of course parents cannot but feel overjoyed by obvious improvements in their child's comfort and well-being. To see such improvements as significant and to rejoice at them does not mean you are being unrealistic or 'failing to come to terms' with the situation, with the fact that your child will never get better. You can rejoice simply (or especially) because your child clearly *feels* better.

We are lucky to have a lot of really good friends and their love and support has helped us immensely. Yet our relationships with our friends were not without pain and tension, particularly in the early stages of Helen's illness. Because of our friendship with them, because we cared about them just as they cared about us, we felt the need to help our friends, to reassure them that we were all right, to help them to relax in our company and not worry about upsetting us by ill-chosen words or unfortunate remarks. We often felt for our friends almost as much as they were undoubtedly feeling for us. At times it was quite exhausting.

I remember one occasion during the first summer after Helen became ill. We had all four been invited to go to tea with good friends who lived in the country, a couple with a baby the same age as Catherine. It was the first time the husband had seen Helen in her helpless state. He was clearly deeply affected by her condition (though he told me later that his wife, who had come to visit Helen, had 'tried to prepare him for it'). As we carried Helen into the garden he started to pour lavish praise on the summer dress she was wearing. It *was* a pretty dress but did not merit the effusive remarks he made about it. We understood his shock at seeing Helen and the fear of hurting us by a stunned silence which made him cast around for something positive to say. Any pain he felt at not knowing what to say or do we shared in rich measure.

In a real friendship the desire and need to give is quite as great as the desire and need to receive. Our need to give was in no way diminished just because we had been, to quote a friend, 'clobbered by fate'. We were of course in great need of help and support, both moral and practical. Yet it is demoralizing and makes you acutely aware of the imbalance in your friendship (which over a long period can be fatal), if you are always *asking*, whether for practical assistance or for a listening ear. The friends who came forward spontaneously, whether with offers to babysit or bearing cakes or other dishes they'd made, or simply to have a drink and a talk about anything and everything with us, were a lifeline. Incidentally, in situations like the one we found ourselves in, it is not pride which stops you asking for help as often as you need it, nor an inability to ask for what you need; it is a fear of gradually eroding a friendship you value by destroying the delicate balance between giving and receiving which underpins all true friendship.

As Helen gradually 'thawed out' at home and became much calmer, so the weather moved from icy winter to mild spring. In the late spring and early summer we would sometimes carry little Helen out into the garden and stretch her out on a mattress in the fresh air, hoping that the natural sounds and smells of the garden would somehow reach her. That year our garden was awash with forget-me-nots (the forget-me-not later became the symbol of Helen House) which grew particularly thickly around the area where Helen had played the previous summer. We had not planted forget-me-nots nor ever had any in the garden; the wind or the birds had done a beautiful (though poignant) propagation job! We began to take Helen out on occasions; though she was not calm or relaxed enough to attend Catherine's christening, performed by her much-loved grand-father in our local church, she was relaxed enough on the day a friend's son was christened to be taken to the christening tea, where she lay peacefully, like Sleeping Beauty, on a sofa. We continued to try to pick up the, at times rather slippery, threads of our 'normal' life.

While Helen was in hospital we had often felt that Helen the person was largely obscured by Helen the medical case, as was perhaps inevitable in such a clinical setting 'programmed' to medical ends. After we brought Helen home we felt it was now we, as much as Helen, who were viewed rather simplistically as 'the case' by those in authority or simply in a position to help. We felt we were seen as the textbook item 'parents of a very sick child' (as though all parents of sick children are the same!) I think it is fair to describe the attitude of health professionals and social workers to us in this way; there was no real approach to us as people but rather an attempt (destined to be at best unhelpful, at worst disastrous) at remote control (or perhaps classification is a better word here) of a case. Shortly after Helen came home we learnt, unofficially and after the event, that a case conference had been held to discuss Helen and us and to 'co-ordinate' the 'official approach' to 'our case'. Our GP was not present at the case conference. Only one of the many people gathered around the table had ever met Helen or us. It was she who, shocked by the time and money wasted in totally uninformed discussion (which of course did not result in any action) relayed the proceedings to us. It was as though Helen's becoming seriously ill had transformed us overnight from individuals with particular characters, interests, tastes and attitudes, into an item in a category. Sometimes it seemed hard to hold on to our identity and individuality.

Because something terrible has happened in your life it does not mean that you as an individual suddenly shed all your previous tastes and interests. It may well be harder to pursue them but they remain. Your personality and interests, likes and dislikes remain fundamentally unchanged; though you often have different and frighteningly new and unfamiliar practical burdens and problems (and could do with some help with these) you remain, as an individual, essentially the same.

A House Called Helen

Perhaps two anecdotes best illustrate what I know others in our situation have experienced. Soon after we brought Helen home from hospital, while we were still struggling to organize ourselves into some semblance of a routine and while we were in a state of disorientating exhaustion, the telephone rang one evening and a woman I had never met and never heard of told me she was ringing to ask me to go Scottish dancing with her. She said she had been given my name and telephone number by someone who worked for the Health Authority and had been told that, like her, I'd got a disabled daughter. She loved Scottish dancing and therefore was sure I would too. It was impossible to tell her bluntly that all-ladies Scottish dancing was not something I'd ever felt drawn to and just because Helen had suddenly been taken ill it did not mean I suddenly felt the urge to try it. She was undoubtedly well-intentioned but it was a wearisome business; she had my phone number and did not hesitate to use it on several occasions. She probably suffered from the abortive phone calls as much as I did; she had been put in touch with me because I was a similar case to her.

One day, in the course of conversation with a nurse, we said we were planning to go to a concert a few days later. 'Oh *good*', came the quick response. 'That'll do you good'. Useless to explain that we were going to the concert because we wanted to go to a concert, we'd always enjoyed going to concerts, we were going for fun. Somehow the outing we had been looking forward to suddenly seemed like some sort of calculated and dreary therapy; the fun of it had evaporated under the force of the conviction with which the nurse stressed its therapeutic benefit to us.

Because we were now 'a case', 'people with a problem', a surprising number of people suddenly felt free to give us unsolicited advice, to comment on just about every aspect of our life, on all sorts of private things. These ranged from our sex life to whether we 'ought to' (in *their* eyes) have another child (whether we wanted one seemed hardly relevant to those who were most enthusiastic in weighing up the theoretical

50

benefits or drawbacks!) At a later date, when I was expecting our third child, an 'official visitor' to our house one day left a card about an anti-abortion group on our sitting room table. Perhaps she thought that Richard and I might, given the enormous stresses and strains of our life, decide to have our much-wanted baby aborted. Somehow, because you have a problem, it is felt that your life is in some way public property; all sorts of sensitive areas can boldly be approached, all sorts of private matters can, with impunity, be dragged under the spotlight. There seemed to us to be a baffling imbalance between the quite startling readiness to discuss our *supposed* emotions and difficulties and the dispiriting reluctance to help us with the glaringly *obvious* practical problems.

Sometimes, indeed, it seems almost as though the abstract discussion provides a useful distraction from the practical problems, a pleasant alternative to getting to grips with what needs to be done. Much later, in a sleep-deprived state and having waited three quarters of an hour for a Health Authority physiotherapist to turn up for an appointment she had requested with me at Helen's special school, I was reduced to tears of frustration by the gross inadequacy of the physiotherapy provision for children like Helen in Oxfordshire. The physiotherapist, seeing my tears, leaned towards me conspiratorially and asked, 'Now tell me, what is *really* the problem?'

It is often said that time is a great healer. We found that our pain at Helen's condition, our feeling of bereavement, actually increased as time went on. With every day that passed we were further away from the lively, vibrant little Helen we had once known. We felt something akin to panic at the idea of losing touch with that little being. We sought out those who had known and loved Helen during her 'well life' and who could, and indeed liked to, talk about her. Fortunately these were many and we never tired of hearing them talk about Helen. The lock-keeper from Abingdon Lock, two elderly neighbours who had doted on Helen, the teacher of Helen's

51

nursery music class, the woman who sold us our milk tokens in the Co-op, the then vicar of Abingdon, a member of our church congregation who had admired Helen's singing – they all, by their oft-repeated reminiscences, provided us with a treasured link with the Helen we had once known, with a past we could not bear to think of as past.

Throughout all this time, Frances was a frequent and very welcome visitor to our home. She shared both our satisfaction as Helen gradually relaxed in her home surroundings and became peaceful and, at the same time, our pain as we realized that this still, quiet creature we nursed was our only link with the vibrant little person we had once known. Frances saw too our increasing exhaustion. She knew about our sad visit to Bradwell Grove. One day, about three months after we had brought Helen home from hospital, Frances asked us if we trusted her enough to 'lend her' Helen for a weekend; she would love to nurse Helen and look after her while we had a short break. We knew how much Frances loved Helen; we knew that she knew how we cared for her and was familiar with the little personal rituals by which that caring was supported. On Helen's behalf we accepted Frances's invitation to her to go and stay with her for a few days in her room in the convent. We dismantled Helen's cot and re-assembled it in the Reverend Mother's private room; we packed Helen's teddy, her mobile, her tape recorder and music tapes, her special blanket – and, of course her drugs, special spoons, nappies and clothes. Helen went to stay with Frances.

We went for a long weekend in Devon with baby Catherine. We rested, enjoyed unbroken nights of sleep and got drunk on fresh air and Catherine's intoxicating, undiluted company. We returned home refreshed.

The seed of Helen House had been sown.

3

Frances and Helen

Helen House is often described as having sprung from friendship, a friendship between a nun and a very ill child and her family. The nature of this friendship was a vital factor in determining what was to arise from it. Our friendship with Frances was a friendship with roots in many shared attitudes and feelings, a friendship nourished by mutual interest and love and by a similar approach to people and events. It was because its roots extended below and beyond the particular tragedy which enveloped our existence at that time that our friendship was able to bear such fruit.

In the early weeks of Helen's illness, which then stretched into months and years, Frances was a frequent visitor to our home. We discussed all sorts of things, not by any means all related to the situation we found ourselves in. We talked about our jobs and why we each did what we did. We talked about our families, about music, about gardens and travel and books we had read. We talked about the Established Church and about the Society of All Saints of which Frances was then the Reverend Mother. We introduced Frances to some of our friends and she brought friends of hers to meet us in our home. We learnt much about Frances's background and about how she had come to be a nun.

Frances was born in Scotland in 1942, the daughter and first child of Norman Ritchie, a chartered accountant, and his wife Peggy, a professional musician. Her parents were living in Inverness at the time of her birth because her father was serving with the London Scottish Regiment whose staff headquarters were there. When Frances was two weeks old she and her mother went to Greenock to live with her mother's parents.

Her mother's mother died when Frances was three weeks old and Frances and her mother then lived with her mother's father in Greenock until the end of the war. Frances says that her family model was a mother, grandfather and child. She saw little of her father but developed a close attachment to her grandfather whom she missed acutely when she and her parents moved south in 1946 to settle near London.

Her early education is not a time Frances looks back on with any enthusiasm; in fact she remembers being very unhappy when she first started going to school because she found the social mixing and 'jollity' difficult. However, soon after she started school she had something to look forward to; her mother was expecting her second child and Frances was very excited at the idea of having a brother or a sister. However, when David was born he was very sick; he was born with only one lung and the doctors were not optimistic about his chances of survival. The first six months of his life were spent in Great Ormond Street Hospital and were anxious times for all the family. David suffered three bouts of pneumonia and on several occasions seemed to cling to life by a mere thread. Inevitably, Frances's mother was absent a great deal of the time as she needed to be with her little son, and Frances saw little of her.

Miraculously, David survived those first stormy months of life and at the age of six months he was strong enough to be taken home. Frances was very involved in her little brother's care when he came home from hospital. She *loved* nursing David; she remembers finding the elaborate precautions the family had to take against infection exciting (she loved donning a mask!) and even derived satisfaction from the mundane and supposedly off-putting tasks that had to be done, such as mopping up sick. She says that she had always, from as far back as she can remember, wanted to nurse; in her games all her dolls were always ill and, incidentally, never got better.

It was David's spell in Great Ormond Street Hospital that made Frances decide that she would like to train there to become a nurse. Her mother's reaction, on Frances's deciding that she would like to take up nursing, was significant: 'Why not medicine?' she asked. Frances's mother can in many ways be seen as something of a pioneer. She had studied music at Somerville College, Oxford and at the Royal College of Music and before the war, in what was still, in terms of career prospects and equal opportunities, very much a man's world, she founded an orchestra of which she was the principal conductor for two and a half years, until the war forced the orchestra to disperse. After the war she was for some years the Chairman of the Society of Women Musicians but there is no doubt that the war, coming when it did, effectively put paid to her hopes of a full-blown musical career. The blighting of her personal ambitions was a cruel blow; perhaps she transferred some of her ambition to her daughter Frances. Certainly, her powerful personality, her determination, her belief that satisfaction stems from achievement in public life and that everybody should strive to realize their full potential were later to colour her reaction to the direction Frances's life was to take.

Having decided that nursing was the career for her, Frances was anxious to become a nurse as soon as possible. She did not enjoy her school days; she felt impatient at school, seeing it as marking time until she could embark on her chosen career. Furthermore, she felt that success at school seemed to go hand-in-hand with being extrovert and she was, at that stage, reserved, shy and lacking in confidence. The fact that her early school days were punctuated by ill health did not help. As a child she contracted tuberculosis for which three months of bed rest and three months' convalescence were prescribed. She remembers the 'cosy times' of illness at home, of being told stories by her father, of being cosseted and of feeling loved and secure. Her brief stays in hospital she found, by contrast, unsettling; interestingly, she says this was because, although the medical care was excellent, the impersonal atmosphere in hospital was intimidating. She describes feeling totally alone

one day as she lay in her hospital bed and thinking, 'There's no one around who knows me or wants to know me'.

The six years she spent at Cheltenham Ladies' College she describes as six years of feeling a failure despite the fact that she had a few good friends. She felt a 'non-person', she did not feel valued. It was only in her last year that she was able to feel any sense of achievement. In this year she embarked on a course in citizenship, designed for the less academically orientated, the non-A level candidates. The course focused on matters of social concern and our approach to them. For the first time in her school career Frances felt she was studying and thinking about matters that were of some relevance to her and what she hoped to do in life. At the end of the course she was awarded a distinction and her work was described as 'quite exceptional'.

Frances left school when she was seventeen. The plan was that she would have a year off before starting her nursing training at eighteen. She spent most of this year at St Hilda's East, a settlement in east London established and supported by her old school. Basically, the idea behind the settlement was that a group of students and professional people working in London would set up home together in a socially-deprived area, providing a solid presence in that area and a focus from which to provide help, advice and facilities for the local people. Frances went in to St Hilda's East on a daily basis, two or three days a week. She got to know the people who came to the settlement for advice and practical help and took part in the activities of the various clubs. She was particularly involved with the Children's Country Holiday Fund and one of her jobs was to go around collecting holiday money (3d a week) from the families living in the tenement blocks around the settlement.

In September 1961 the day Frances had been looking forward to for years arrived; she began her nurse's training at Great Ormond Street Hospital. She believed she was at last embarking on something she really could do and she was filled with new confidence. Her social life blossomed; she lived in the nurses' home and made many friends. She was selected to do the comprehensive training leading to the two qualifications of RSCN and SRN and she speaks of the next four years, divided between Great Ormond Street and the Middlesex Hospitals, as very happy.

While at the Middlesex, Frances nursed a man who spent six weeks in the hospital following a coronary. She knew he was a priest because of his name – the Reverend Dick Chamberlin – but she assumed, wrongly, that he was a Roman Catholic because of the stream of nuns and cassocked clergy who visited him and 'the books with coloured ribbon markers' on his locker. When he left hospital, the Reverend Dick Chamberlin invited Frances to go to tea with him, an invitation she did not take up. However, when he returned to the hospital as an out-patient he repeated his invitation to Frances to go and visit him some time and this time she did. He lived in the clergy house next to his church which was an extreme Anglo-Catholic establishment. He took Frances to see his church, which struck her as unusually ornate, and introduced her to the team of people connected with his ministry, three sisters and two curates. Frances soon started attending services at the church regularly.

Although she cannot recall a time when she was not aware of having a personal relationship with God, organized religion had not played a very important part in Frances's early life. Her grandfather, whom she adored, was an Elder of the Church of Scotland and she had attended church with him and later, as many children do, she had gone to Sunday School. At Cheltenham Ladies' College, church attendance was compulsory. Frances resisted early confirmation though she was later confirmed at the age of sixteen. Before she met Dick Chamberlin, Frances says that any religious leanings she had, had been towards orders such as the Quakers; she felt most at home with simplicity in worship. Her heroines were people like Elizabeth Fry, that is to say social reformers whose religious commitment was the background to their pioneering work in the wider community.

However, her introduction to Dick Chamberlin opened a new world; it revealed to Frances whole new dimensions to faith and worship. She was drawn into a world of spirituality fed and sustained by regular worship. For the first time in her life she felt part of that worship.

During the last year of her nursing training Frances took lodgings with one of Dick Chamberlin's parishioners and became ever more involved with his church. Following a parish outing to Walsingham in 1964 she says she suddenly knew that she had to try her vocation in a religious community. She told Dick Chamberlin of her conviction and was slightly surprised when he told her to 'go away and forget it'. The simplicity and single-mindedness of religious commitment appealed to Frances very strongly and she was impatient to make such a commitment herself. Dick Chamberlin, however, felt she should beware of acting impulsively. 'If in a year's time you feel the same, come back,' he told her. 'If your vocation is genuine, it will not go away.'

Looking back, Frances says that it was at this stage that she made a big mistake. She told her parents of her intention to join a religious order. They were horrified, seeing Frances's plan as, at best, a ridiculous but passing romantic whim and, at worst, a total waste of her life. Her parents' strong disapproval compounded the pain Frances felt at the idea of giving up nursing and her last months at Great Ormond Street were stressful. The atmosphere at home when Frances visited her family was tense – very different from the happiness that had pervaded the carefree weekends and holidays of her childhood. Her father was repelled by the idea of his only daughter joining a religious order but, having made his views clear, chose not to talk about it. By contrast, her mother talked about it at every possible opportunity, expressing her contempt for Frances's proposed future forcefully and untiringly. Frances's brother David occasionally sought refuge from the tension at home with a family in Reigate to whom he was introduced by a friend of his mother. Ironically, it was through his acquaintance with this family and everything that this led to, that David was later to be ordained. His ordination and ministry, however, never caused any ructions in the Ritchie family. A vicar has, after all, a recognized and widely-appreciated role in public life and is very much part of the social order. Furthermore, of course, a Church of England vicar can marry and have children. David's faith never caused him the acute problems *vis-à-vis* his parents that Frances's was to cause her.

Nine months after the parish outing to Walsingham Frances returned to Dick Chamberlin. Despite her parents' hostility, she had not wavered in her conviction that life in a religious community was what she was destined for. After a long talk with Dick Chamberlin, she asked if she could go and visit a few convents and, because he knew it well, Dick Chamberlin arranged for her to go and visit All Saints at London Colney. As she walked up the drive to the convent house, Frances knew that she was, literally and metaphorically, on the right path.

The Mother Superior General of the Order of All Saints was at that time Mother Catherine. Talking to her and feeling her understanding and support was very soothing to Frances after the bitter outpourings of her family. It was Mother Catherine who insisted that Frances should not only complete her training at Great Ormond Street but also make up the seven months she had missed at the hospital through recurrence of her earlier health problems. Having done this, Frances then went to give help in the house to family friends in Grimsby for six weeks, and then for a holiday with her great friend from her nursing days who now lived in Denmark. These changes of scene and contact with different life styles did nothing to undermine her conviction that life in a religious community was for her.

On 6th July 1966 Frances entered the Society of All Saints as a postulant. Life as a postulant involved living and worshipping with the community without actually being part of it. As Frances puts it, postulants were 'let in gently'. During this trial period the postulant is closely observed by the Mother Superior, the Novice Guardian and the Chaplain General who then debate her suitability for the next stage. On 16th November 1966 Frances was clothed as a novice. She received her habit; for the last four and a half months she had worn the postulant's home-made black frock with white collar and veil. With the habit the novice wore a leather belt, a white ivory cross and a starched wimple and veil. As a novice, Frances was integrated a little more into the community but remained under the tutelage of the Novice Mistress (nowadays called the Guardian) who was in charge of her spiritual development and day-to-day welfare. Frances received instructions in such subjects as Liturgy, Spirituality and Prayer. She worked in the kitchen and cleaning the chapel and also worked part-time in the small children's home run by the community, which she loved. She remained a novice until April 1969.

Before that date, however, the serious illness of her aunt-by-marriage drew Frances out of the community for five months. She moved in to the home of her father's brother and nursed his wife for the last few days of her life. She then stayed on in their home for several months in order to help provide some sort of secure and ordered existence for her two young cousins. During this period she inevitably came into contact with her own immediate family again. They made no secret of the fact that they hated seeing her in her habit and 'worked on her' to leave the community. They were devastated when Frances returned to London Colney.

Frances took vows for three years on 16th April 1969. When, on 20th April 1972, she took her life vows, she was unsupported by her family, but a good number of friends and well-wishers came to be with her on what was the greatest day of her life. These included the Principal of Cheltenham Ladies' College and the Matron of Great Ormond Street Hospital.

For many years Frances was emotionally, if not literally, an orphan. Her family virtually disowned her on her becoming a nun. Although she is characteristically generous, forgiving and non-judgemental in her attempts to understand her family's (and more especially her mother's) attitude towards her, the harshness of their treatment and the pain it caused her cannot be overstated. As a postulant and novice, Frances received 'threatening' letters from her mother warning her of the dire consequences her selfish behaviour would have; it would break up her parents' marriage, it would kill her adored grandfather, it would make David fail his exams. Her mother urged her to consider her position as Frances's mother; how could she explain things to her friends? She was unremitting in her desperate attempts to make Frances change her mind.

Sometimes her mother changed tack and urged Frances to think of the career she might have had in nursing. Why was she considering walling herself up and not using her talents? Couldn't she channel her 'vocation' to serve into something more socially acceptable? Sue Ryder and others were held up to Frances as role models. Her mother saw nuns' spirituality as introspective, self-indulgent and unrelated to the needs of the world. She could not grasp the idea of God's call which, as Frances explains, when you have heard it once, you follow unquestioningly or you have no peace of mind. Moreover, you follow the call not knowing where it will take you. Later, Helen House was to Frances an unlooked-for bonus in her life of dedication; the possibility of a commitment to the religious life enabling you to develop your practical skills in a field very dear to you would never be a sound basis, in Frances's eyes, on which to make that commitment. By contrast, in Frances's mother's eyes you could not be drawn to something as nebulous as spirituality; you looked first at the outward manifestations, the fruits, of that spirituality. If these were not very obviously beneficial to the world then there was no point in embracing that spirituality.

Frances's mother's hostility to the religious life and her rejection of her daughter when she chose to embrace it perhaps had much to do with her own thwarted professional career.

Perhaps the dashing of her own hopes had caused her such cruel disappointment as to make her wish to protect her daughter from similar pain? It is significant that, though Frances remains a nun, her mother is now fully reconciled to the religious life her daughter has chosen and indeed both her parents are now keen and loving supporters both of Frances and of the hospice she has founded. The acceptance of Frances's chosen life style and the healing of the rift between mother and daughter came when Helen House was planned and Frances became known as its founder, with all the public acclaim and recognition that went with this. Suddenly Frances had a career and appeared to be realizing her potential in the public forum.

Looking back on her early days as a nun, Frances says that she was deeply happy but bore the continuing pain of knowing she had hurt those she loved. Her spiritual gifts were quickly recognized within the Society. In August 1975 she was asked to be the Novice Mistress and she worked in this capacity for about two years. The Novitiate was at this time based in Oxford, the convent at London Colney having been sold in 1973. Until the mid-seventies Oxford had been just a branch house of the Society of All Saints, with about six or eight nuns in residence. Its main purpose had been to run St John's Home, a nursing home for the elderly which had been in existence since 1874. After St John's Home was reduced in size, it became possible for Oxford to become the mother house of the community, which it did in 1976.

In 1977 elections were held for the post of Reverend Mother of the Society of All Saints. At this time the system was that a newcomer to the post was elected for a period of seven years with the possibility of re-election for a further five. The sisters nominate candidates and a secret ballot determines who will occupy the post. In September 1977, when she was only thirty-four and had been in the community for only eleven years, the sisters elected Frances Mother Superior General, a position she was to occupy for twelve years until 1989.

Frances feels that the confidence the sisters placed in her and their strong support drew out qualities in her which she never knew she possessed and helped her conquer the diffidence which had sometimes paralysed her in the past. She set about making adaptations to the convent premises and activities. Hospitality (on a small scale) had always been seen as one of the community's concerns and it was further to translate this concern into action that Frances oversaw the building of the convent guest wing. It was under her supervision that the Bethlehem Chapel, a small simple chapel where the sisters and others can go for prayer and reflection, was built in the convent grounds. It was soon after Frances became Reverend Mother that there was a change in the traditional attire of the nuns; in place of the austere black habits they had previously worn, they began to wear cornflower blue ones. Frances, with the backing of the majority of the sisters, encouraged the sisters to wear mufti on their days off and when they went on holiday.

In a sense, Frances's youth hurried up the 'democratizing process' in the community. Because Frances, the Reverend Mother, was so comparatively young, authority and wisdom were no longer seen as the prerogative of the middle-aged or old. This led to an unleashing of talents and aptitudes hitherto unsuspected; everyone, young and old, felt that they had something to contribute, a part to play.

It had been the vision of the Mother Foundress, Harriet Brownlow Byron, that the Society of All Saints should work with children. From the outset, the sisters of the community had worked with orphans and in 1883 they founded the Bradford Hospital for the Children of the Poor. This was to ensure that sick children from very poor families received the treatment and care they needed if they were to recover. In addition to their work with sick children in Bradford, the community also worked in the early days with convalescent children in Eastbourne. After the death of the Mother Foundress in 1887, a decision was made to build a Convalescent Children's Hospital in her memory. This hospital was called St Luke's and was opened on 19th July 1890 by the Prince and Princess of Wales, accompanied by the Princesses Victoria and Maud.

The fact that Frances should have got to know Helen when she did, particularly since, as I have said before, our original meeting was so dependent on chance, was an extraordinary coincidence, some might say a miracle. At the time Frances met Helen, the community was becoming aware of the deliberations and decrees emanating from the second Vatican Council. One of the things that was being said to members of religious communities was that they should strive to return to the charism (vision) of their founder. It was felt that many congregations had 'gone off the boil' because they had been unfaithful to the original vision that fuelled them. To seek to return to that original vision did not mean clinging blindly and unquestioningly to tradition, but rather seeking to adapt tradition to suit modern times. Frances's meeting with Helen and the close friendship which quickly grew up between us and all that arose from that, could hardly have happened at a more appropriate time in the life of the community. The work of Helen House is very much in accord with the original vision of their Foundress and being involved in its foundation meant that the sisters of All Saints were indeed returning to their spiritual roots.

Frances appeared to us to be the perfect embodiment of the dual role of the community she headed, the practical and the spiritual, which find their expression in work and prayer. She was uniquely able to help us and be the friend we needed because, as I saw it, her feet were planted firmly on the ground but her head was in heaven! Imprisoned as we often felt in the tragedy which had overtaken us and all its attendant problems, we desperately needed, as we looked through the bars of our prison, to see the stars as well as the mud. Frances helped us to keep on doing this. Those who saw Helen in purely physical terms were bound to see her now as simply a burden and we could not bear to see our beloved daughter so diminished. Incidentally, some of those people who saw Helen as merely a burden did little to help us carry that burden. (I must include here the 'caring services'; getting help, equipment or simply information about how or where to get help, equipment or benefits from 'the professionals' continued to be a time-consuming struggle.) Frances shared our feeling that Helen's spirit was not quenched by her physical impairment. Of course she was not blind to Helen's physical impairment and total helplessness, but she helped us with the burden of caring for Helen without ever defining Helen herself as that burden. Frederick Langbridge[1] suggests that as you look through the bars you see *either* mud *or* stars; surely, though, seeing the mud does not stop you raising your eyes to the stars; in fact, I would suggest, you *need* to raise your eyes to the stars in order to cope with the mud.

Helen herself, from the moment she was born, had led us to 'see the stars'. We had always known that we wanted children but we were quite unprepared for the strength of the love, wonderment and joy that Helen awakened in us. Parenthood took us by storm – and very delightful it was to be thus conquered! Being parents was a totally positive experience for us. It seems odd that babies (and children generally) are most often described in terms of the negative or disruptive impact they have, or do not have, on their parents' lives. Thus a baby is said to be 'good' if she doesn't wake her parents in the night or doesn't regurgitate her feed, not because she has done something positive to enhance her parents' lives. Helen brought so much to our lives. We delighted in her company; her presence complemented our existing closeness and happiness. She was a remarkably happy little person with a rather strange self-containment. At a very tender age she showed an adult concern for others and was clearly troubled by anxiety or ill-ease in others. A basic instinct towards

[1] 'Two men look out through prison bars, One sees the mud, the other stars.' *Frederick Langbridge*

happiness seemed to make her feel that this was the natural state for everyone. She loved music and had a very controlled, clear and tuneful singing voice; not many two-year-olds are singled out as potential choristers by members of the church congregation! She loved going into churches and early town walks and country drives were punctuated by visits to churches of all kinds. 'I happy here', she once explained as I sat in a pew waiting for her to complete her peregrinations around the aisles. Perhaps the fact that her much-loved grandfather was a vicar and she would go with him to his church and watch him wind the clock, or would potter around while he emptied collecting boxes or sorted books, had something to do with this.

One day Helen announced her plans for the future. 'When I big I play the cello', she told us. We treasure a letter from a music teacher telling us she thought Helen was musically gifted and that she felt she could 'do something for her'. We have many tapes and discs of cello music which we play to Helen as she lies on her bean bag; we like to think the mellow sound of the instrument she had set her heart on playing touches that heart with joy.

Helen quite simply enhanced our already happy life and shed light on us. The letters we received when she was so suddenly taken ill (and have continued to receive) testify to the way she touched the lives of others too. No aspect of life with Helen ever seemed burdensome to us. We were perhaps, in some people's eyes, besotted; we certainly never felt that Helen's presence was in any way a constraint on our lives. Where we had previously been two we were now three. One of the most shocking aspects of Helen's sudden illness was that until she was taken into hospital I had never spent a night under a different roof from her.

I realize that even after we had been told that Helen had no chance of recovery, hope still lingered obstinately within us and the belief that we might recapture those halcyon days with 'well' Helen refused to be driven out. It was, I suppose, this hope and belief, coupled with what was presumably a belief that Frances had her head very much in heaven, that made me feel that we might come home to find Helen miraculously cured after her first weekend stay with Frances. I was not aware that I had believed this to be possible until, on the way back from our weekend break in Devon, we stopped in Newbury to ring Frances and to tell her we were nearly home. I remember the huge wave of disappointment that swept over me as I stood in the telephone box when, in answer to my questions about Helen, Frances told me she was fine, she had slept well and taken her drugs and food well and had not been unduly disturbed. I suddenly realized I had packed a particular dress in Helen's case because I had thought she would look so good in it, skipping out to meet us on our return.

A basic instinct for survival makes most of us hold fast to hope against all odds and act under its impulse, for without hope we cannot go forward. Hope is not necessarily sustained by logic or reason, by belief in the possibility of what you hope for, but equally logic and reason cannot quench it. We had experienced this very powerfully while Helen was still in hospital. Although I knew from the day of her operation that Helen would not recover, I was able to work to help her get better with a total conviction that recovery was just around the corner. A passage from *Incline our Hearts* by A. N. Wilson analyses very well this ability to operate at two seemingly contradictory levels:

> It was an example of that touching human propensity to behave as though there were a future even when reason declares that there isn't. The man on his walk to the gallows asks permission to stoop down and tie his shoelace. The Jewish woman brushes mud off her husband's shoulder in the queue for the gas ovens, though clothes (muddy or otherwise) and life itself are soon to be surrendered. These are not the actions of foolish optimists. Rather, instinct keeps them straining

towards the sun, even when they no longer believe in the future.

Incline our Hearts, A. N. Wilson

Straining towards the sun was, I suppose, what we were doing when we took Helen to healing services, though some might call it clutching at straws. Richard and I had to quash our intellectual qualms about taking part in such services, which in normal circumstances would have been considerable. The fact that we were able to do so is an indication, perhaps, of our desperation, of our need to clutch at straws. Equally, it could be an example of the 'touching human propensity to behave as though there were a future when reason declares there isn't', which A. N. Wilson refers to.

Whatever our motives, Frances and I drove Helen miles, in raw early spring weather, to attend a healing service in Essex conducted by the Reverend Trevor Dearing. Later, we attended a similar service in Swindon. They were strange occasions where the feeling of warmth, fellowship and mutual support that pervaded the gathering – whether manufactured or genuine it matters little – were almost palpable.

Another instance of the power of hope over the evidence supplied (often in ample measure, too) by reason and observation, is to be found in Richard's letters to Hilary, the nursery nurse who helped us with Helen at home. Looking back at the letters Richard wrote at the end of each month when he sent Hilary a cheque to pay for her wonderful work with Helen, we find sentences such as, 'We are still working towards a complete recovery.' Wild hope is not the province simply of those who undervalue the intellect.

The seed of Helen House was sown, as I have said, on that first occasion when Helen went to stay with Frances for a long weekend while we had a break. One day about six months later, Frances rang and asked if she could come over and talk about something with us. As we sat together in our sitting room, with Helen lying on a mattress between us, she told us

that she had begun to feel she would like to help other families
in rather the same way as she helped us. Being involved with
Helen and with us and seeing all the problems that confronted
us had made her realize how little support was available for
families in our situation and, moreover, had revived in her a
long-buried wish she had cherished in her nursing days when
she had longed to establish some sort of home for ill children.
Reviving this idea fitted in very well with her present desire
to extend the work of the Society of All Saints in the wider
community. We sat and talked and as we talked a rough picture
began to emerge of how Frances's idea might take concrete
form.

Some sort of place would be set up which would help families
looking after a very ill child at home by offering them
friendship, practical and moral support and, most important,
respite care for their very ill child for short periods, to enable
them to recharge their batteries and summon up the strength
to carry on with the exhausting job of caring for their child.
The place would be small and homely, non-institutional, non-
medical, and as unlike a hospital as possible; the emphasis
would be on the child as a person.

As it happened there was a potential site where the place
we were beginning to picture in our minds, still somewhat
hazily, might be built. At the far end of the gardens of All Saints
Convent, beyond the more formal area, was a largish area of
land which was fairly overgrown and not much used, except
by the sisters when they sought extra quiet and isolation. If
the sisters were agreeable (the convent operates on very
democratic principles) it might be possible to use this land to
build on. Moreover, this would in some ways be in the interests
of the community since Oxford City Council had noted the
existence of the 'very extensive' grounds of St John's Home
and had in fact written in 1968 to ask if there were any
'likelihood of the Order being prepared to enter into negotiation
to sell the land' as a site for a new primary school in East
Oxford.

In addition, the Senior Medical Officer from the City of Oxford Health Department had written in 1973 to put forward the possibility of the development of the land to provide new housing for the elderly. Although the Mother Superior had responded to both enquiries by explaining that the Society of All Saints did not wish at that time either to expand their work with the elderly beyond what they felt confident they could do to a very high standard, or to sell any of their land in Oxford, the enquiries inevitably focused the community's thoughts on how the land was, and should be, used. If it could be used in a way which would so obviously benefit families and children in great need, this should be to everyone's satisfaction.

It began suddenly to seem to us as though the tragedy that had befallen Helen were really meant to lead to something very positive. Things seemed to be falling into place (to our eager eyes, anyway) remarkably naturally. Interestingly, this feeling was to grow, not to evaporate, over the months that followed, as our plans took shape. People talk of 'accidents waiting to happen'; we soon came to feel that Helen House (as it was to become) was a dream waiting to be realized. Without belittling the enormous efforts of a huge number of people who were to identify with our project, or minimizing the practical hurdles that had to be cleared, I can say that we felt we were carried along on a natural tide, that things somehow fell into place. It may sound fanciful to say this, but it was as though Helen was the 'enabler' of some preordained scheme.

From that first conversation with Frances in our home about her desire to help other families in similar situations to our own by building some sort of hospice or haven, we felt hugely enthusiastic about the idea. What we did not know was how great the need was for the place we envisaged. We had no idea how many families, locally and indeed country-wide, were caring for very ill children at home without the back-up of respite care and practical support. Before proceeding further, we felt we should try to gauge the need. I rang up Helen's

70

neurosurgeon and arranged for Frances and myself to go and see him. He was very supportive of the project we outlined to him and told us that he believed there were many families who would benefit from the sort of service we hoped to establish. He urged us to press on with our scheme. We left feeling we must now proceed to action!

Frances then consulted other doctors and nurses and paediatricians to obtain their opinions. In particular, she talked of her idea to Roger Burne, a GP with the East Oxford Health Centre which served the convent and also the old people's home attached to the convent. He was keenly interested in the scheme and offered ideas of his own as to how a hospice for sick children might operate. We, too, talked the idea over with friends from both medical and non-medical backgrounds and gathered opinions. On Friday 28th March 1980 a small meeting was convened in Mother Frances's room at All Saints Convent, where on several occasions now she had welcomed Helen to stay for a few days. The stated purpose of that meeting was 'to discuss the foundation of a hospice for severely sick children – "Helen House".'

We never looked back.

4

Planning the Hospice

That first meeting on 28th March 1980 and a subsequent one two months later laid the foundations for the translation of an idea into reality. The people who attended those early meetings were not a committee but rather, I would say, a committed group. We had not been appointed to serve because of paper qualifications or our standing in society. We were all keenly interested in the idea of a children's hospice and had something definite to contribute to its planning. We were united by a common purpose and a positive determination to act.

Our discussions had a very clear focus. Frances has often commented on Helen's vital role in our deliberations; Helen, her plight and our life caring for her, the things that eased or alternatively aggravated our problems, the type of support and care we and Helen needed and, above all, the quality of care we wanted for Helen at all times, whether at home or elsewhere, provided the model for what a purpose-built children's hospice would offer other children and their families. To start from the particular and familiar and work outwards often works better than trying to hone down the general and make it successful in particular circumstances.

The people present at that first meeting in March 1980 were:

Mother Frances Dominica (Reverend Mother, All Saints Convent),
Dr Roger Burne (GP),
John Bicknell (Architect),
Derreck Shorten (Architectural Consultant),
Bronwen Bennett (Physiotherapist),
Vivien Pritchard (Nursing Officer at Sir Michael Sobell House),

Sister Margaret (Society of All Saints) and
Richard Worswick (Helen's father).

Michael Briggs (Consultant Neurosurgeon), David Paterson
(Accountant), and Jacqueline Worswick apologised for being
unable to attend. Richard and I alternated at meetings, one
of us attending each time while the other looked after Helen
and Catherine.

Richard describes the atmosphere at the start of that first
meeting as being one of quiet expectation, of awe almost.
A pin dropping would have seemed as intrusively noisy in
the hush that preceded Frances's opening words as a clap of
thunder in less special circumstances. The stillness was broken
by Frances's quiet, sure voice. She began by explaining that
the idea she had harboured for some time of establishing some
sort of hospice for severely sick children had been rekindled
by the plight of Helen. She outlined what had happened to
Helen, how she had first met us shortly after Helen's first,
and major, operation and how our friendship had developed.
She described her visits to Helen in hospital and the several
long weekends Helen had spent with her at All Saints Convent
since returning home in order to give us a short break.

Frances explained that whilst previously she had observed
the workings of children's wards from the staff side, she had
been able, when visiting Helen in hospital, to observe and,
indeed, experience, things from the receiving end. She had
seen how difficult it was for all involved to change from
working towards, and expecting, progressive improvement,
to accepting that a child was not going to recover. With their
high turnover of medical and (usually young) nursing staff,
hospitals were not well-suited to looking after children once
the acute phase of treatment was over. While everyone would
agree that ideally, when acute hospital treatment was complete,
children should be cared for at home, this was not always
possible. Frances felt that there was a need for a hospice which
could care for very sick and dying children and which could

73

provide support of both a practical and spiritual nature for parents and families trying to look after such children at home.

Frances said that she had already discussed her ideas with a number of people, including Mr Briggs (Helen's neuro-surgeon), Dr Baum (a consultant paediatrician) and Dr Robert Twycross, Physician-in-Charge at Sir Michael Sobell House as well as with others among us present at the meeting and she had received considerable, sometimes enthusiastic, support. The group then went on to discuss the desirability of consulting a wider body of opinion at this stage. There was a dilemma here. On the one hand it was important to obtain as wide a range of views as possible and to ensure that the hospice would fit in, and not overlap, with existing services. On the other hand it was important not to over-expose the ideas for the hospice, since that might raise expectations prematurely. It was felt that a forthcoming meeting with a group of hospital paediatricians would be useful in indicating the reaction of local hospital services and it was further agreed that it might also be desirable to consult a number of general practitioners.

One point that has to be stressed is that it was always intended that Helen House should fill a gap in the existing provision. It was never intended that it should set out to be, or should become, a replacement for any existing service. Thus the spirit behind Helen House was totally positive; the wish to establish a children's hospice in no way implied a criticism of any service already available. Helen House was seen as a much-needed addition to the range of services then available to the very ill and those who cared for them.

Having decided to proceed cautiously with consultations, the meeting then moved on to discuss the possible admissions policy for the hospice. Dr Roger Burne circulated some notes he had prepared in which certain criteria for judging suitability for admission were listed. In his view, the hospice was not intended to provide long-term residential care nor to admit children with primary mental handicap. Moreover, it was certainly not intended for children for whom an acute hospital ward would be more suitable. The first claim on the hospice's facilities would come from children in need of terminal care, but children would also be accepted for nursing care to provide family relief for an agreed period (not exceeding, say, four weeks at any one time). Dr Burne also expressed the view that the balance between the probably small number of terminally ill cases and children requiring continuing care, would need further evaluation.

In further, informal, discussions, we later came to the conclusion that of, say, eight beds, six would probably be 'bookable' for respite care, some time in advance if this helped families (for example with holiday arrangements) and two would not be available for such booking. These two would be kept for sudden need, one to allow flexibility – to enable the hospice, for example, to respond to a sudden family crisis which might unexpectedly cause a Helen House family to require relief care for their ill child – and one as an emergency bed, for a child who was suddenly very ill or at the end of his or her life.

The meeting then discussed the key questions of the degree of medical support required at the hospice and medical treatment. It is important to remember in this context that the starting point for Helen House was not a medical one. Helen House arose out of a friendship, a friendship between Frances and Helen and ourselves and the overriding aim of a hospice modelled on Helen's and our needs would be to offer friendship and support for families caring at home for a child whom medical science could not make better. With this clearly in mind it was logical to state that the hospice would not undertake active medical treatment aimed at cure but that it would provide active treatment aimed at pain relief and symptom control.

Children admitted from home for short periods would probably be under the medical supervision of their family GP who would, ideally, continue to supervise his or her patient's treatment during that patient's stay at the hospice. (I should stress here that a child coming to stay at Helen House is never referred to as a patient of Helen House, but as a friend or visitor. The word patient in this context refers to the child's status in relation to his or her GP.) However, it might not always be possible for the GP to continue to supervise the child's treatment while the child was staying at Helen House (the distance between the child's home and Helen House might make this impossible) and in this case the hospice would have to be prepared to assume full medical responsibility. For a terminally-ill child the hospice's medical officer would be even more likely to need to assume responsibility for that child's medical care. Everybody agreed that a very important factor in the successful operation of the planned hospice would be good communications with hospital doctors and GPs. Incidentally, in referring to the hospice's medical officer, nobody envisaged a resident person but rather a doctor whose services would be readily available as and when required. The model for Helen House was the family home, not a hospital.

Discussion then followed on the nursing staff the hospice would require. Even if it had only ten beds (in fact we were to aim higher than this, in terms of quality of care, by having even fewer!) it was felt that, because it would always be necessary to have a trained nurse among those on duty, the hospice would probably need at least ten full-time nursing staff in order to provide twenty-four-hour cover. It was suggested that this core of nursing staff would be supplemented by parents as well as by volunteers from the convent and elsewhere. (In the event, of course, a much higher number of paid staff were employed.) What is perhaps more interesting here than calculations relating to numbers is the fact that it was recognized at an early stage that, wherever they came from, not all the staff who would care for the children needed to be trained nurses, any more than did the relatives, friends and neighbours who probably helped look after that child at home. It was uppermost in our minds all the time that the hospice would provide care for children who were normally looked after at home. Thus it was a temporary substitute for home, not hospital.

When the discussion moved on to the building requirements for the hospice this fact was in the forefront of our minds and shaped our opinions as to what was needed in the way of rooms and facilities. Discussion of the hospice's building requirements centred on some notes prepared by Derreck Shorten. He said that the building should reflect the aim that the hospice should provide care as similar as possible to that provided in a child's home. Probably the majority of children would be accommodated in single rooms, although, as Derreck Shorten explained, it might be possible to have well sound-proofed inter-connecting doors which could be left open in circumstances when children and/or parents developed friendships. This idea met with approval. Flexibility was something everybody felt to be important; from the outset we wished to be able to respond to, and provide for, different attitudes and tastes. The bedrooms need not be identical and should reflect the character of a home with perhaps a pin board for posters etc. Each room should include space for a divan for a parent to sit or sleep on.

It was agreed that there was probably no need for a separate treatment room, although facilities for physiotherapy were of paramount importance. Dr Roger Burne felt that there was no need for a separate consulting room; if and when necessary, doctors would examine children in their own rooms.

The fact that Helen House was aiming to provide a temporary substitute for the child's home led all present to agree that no expensive structural facilities of a medical nature needed to be considered, though obviously portable equipment and aids of various sorts might need to be used to cope with the problems of individual children. John Bicknell and Derreck Shorten explained that, like those in an ordinary home, communal rooms could be multifunctional. They envisaged a short chain of perhaps two or three small rooms for home teaching, play etc., in addition to a central living room. Frances felt that facilities for music were important and Vivien Pritchard spoke of the importance of having one or more quiet rooms where it would be possible for staff to talk to parents in calm and privacy.

This last point led to a discussion of the type and extent of facilities required for parents. Our experience with Helen in hospital had led Richard and me to understand and feel the importance to parents of being able to be with their ill child and yet to withdraw at times to somewhere comfortable, quiet and yet close by. We felt that the single beds/sofas in the children's bedrooms were an excellent idea but felt that further accommodation for parents was needed as well.

The discussion of building requirements ended with a recognition of the obvious need for staff facilities, including perhaps a room for the sister-in-charge. There would also, it was agreed, need to be plenty of storage space for cots, linen, luggage etc. If it was not prohibitively expensive, a small heated pool would be a very pleasant and useful facility.

The meeting ended with a discussion of future plans. Derreck Shorten and John Bicknell explained the customary procedure for projects of this nature. There would need to be a Project Manager – in this case Mother Frances. It would be useful for her to be supported by a working party consisting of a good cross-section of interests. Three phases in the planning process were identified: general agreement of aims, agreement of outline plans, and detailed planning. We agreed that a draft document outlining the philosophy, aims and admissions policy of the hospice should be prepared and discussed with a number of interested parties. The document should be modified if necessary in the light of comments received and should then form the definitive statement of the hospice's aims. The document would be able to provide a rough indication of the hospice's running costs. As soon as this draft document was ready another meeting of our small group would be convened to discuss it and to start considering in detail the schedule of accommodation. John Bicknell would then produce provisional drawings based on the agreed aims and schedule of accommodation. These drawings could form the basis of further discussion and at this stage an approximate capital cost could be estimated. This phase should end in agreement of outline plans which should be formally expressed by the signing of the appropriate documents. Detailed planning would then follow.

On the important subject of money-raising Mother Frances explained that the Society would soon have available to it a large sum (approximately £100,000) which would go some way towards the expected building costs. (These we put very provisionally at about £250,000, excluding furnishings.) It was thought that raising the remaining capital sum would be much easier than providing the continuing running costs which, with a staff of, say, ten, could be very substantial. Frances said that she had already opened an account ('Helen House Account') and that the sum of money in it was already over £50! She mentioned that the Society of All Saints was already a registered charity. Derreck Shorten thought that on completion of phase 1 (the general agreement of aims) it would be possible to produce a brochure describing the proposed hospice and that this could be used for money-raising activities.

At our second meeting, on 16th May 1980, the draft document we had agreed to produce at the end of the first meeting provided the focus for our discussion. This outlined the background to Helen House and gave information about the admissions policy, the organization and staff and the buildings and facilities. It ended with a section on costs and money-raising. Basically, the document was a clear statement of our aims, a distillation of what we had agreed on at our first meeting, with some additional points and details. A few new points had emerged following further reflection on the deliberations at the March meeting and comments from interested parties not present on that occasion.

Under admissions policy, the importance of providing relief nursing care for children with long-term illness, alongside terminal care, was underlined. This relief care would be provided either at regular, agreed intervals for periods not exceeding four weeks or at irregular intervals to enable families to take a holiday or to cover periods of crisis at home. It was stated that the balance between the probably small number of terminally-ill children and those requiring continuing care would obviously vary but an effort would be made to ensure that facilities would always be available for emergency family relief. Contact would be maintained with families between admissions. This, we felt, was very important. Initial referrals for admission would be accepted from consultants, general practitioners or from the family itself. Before admission, contact would be established with the child's medical adviser. Children admitted to Helen House would be in need of substantial nursing care. Children would not normally be admitted over the age of fifteen.

In the discussion at the meeting it was agreed not to write any geographical restriction into the admissions policy at that stage. Because of the importance of easy access for children's families, it was thought likely that children would not come from a great distance. (This, of course, has proved not to be the case.) It was also agreed to make it clear in any brochure or leaflet that children in need of the sort of hospice care Helen House would provide would be welcomed irrespective of race or belief. I like to think that the only entrance qualification for Helen House is need.

Under the heading 'Organization and Staff', it was stated that children admitted to the hospice would be cared for by a team of fully-qualified nurses who would provide twenty-four-hour cover. These nurses would be supported by nursing auxiliaries and volunteers who would include sisters from the Society of All Saints. Physiotherapy, education and play therapy would be provided, where possible, by existing home-visiting services. Members of the child's own family and friends would be encouraged to take an active part in all aspects of the child's care. In the discussion on this section of the document, the importance of continuing education, even in the final stages of illness, was stressed. It is the statutory obligation of the Education Service to provide this for children over the age of five. It was agreed that at a later stage an approach would be made to the LEA to discuss this matter and to discuss liaison with the Home Tuition Service.

The draft document further stated that children admitted from home for short periods would, where possible, continue to be under the medical supervision of their own GP. However, medical cover would be provided by a GP from East Oxford Health Centre who would assume full medical responsibility in appropriate cases. After a lengthy discussion about medical cover, it was agreed that, although the amount of medical support required would vary, it seemed likely that a high percentage of the children would be in a stable condition, not requiring frequent alteration of drug regime or night calls. However, it would be difficult to assess this with any accuracy until the hospice was actually running. Emphasis was placed on the importance of continuity of nursing staff, of having a 'stable hard core'. For this reason reciprocal arrangements with other agencies would not be encouraged and nor would the employment of short-term staff. Richard and I felt very relieved about this. When your child is very ill over a long period of time, it helps enormously to be able to get to know the people involved in treating, or caring for, him or her. Moreover, those people are able to care for your child more sensitively, or simply more efficiently, if they are able to get to know him or her.

The document under discussion further stated that the Society of All Saints would be responsible for the overall policy of the hospice, appointment of staff and financial administration. A sister-in-charge would be responsible for the day-to-day running and administration of the hospice and, in co-operation with the medical officer, would decide on admissions. The meeting decided that the title Head Nurse should be substituted for sister-in-charge in the document and in all discussion in future.

A House Called Helen

On the subject of buildings and facilities, the draft document outlined the main requirements for the hospice agreed on at our March meeting but listed other specific facilities as well. In addition to accommodation of a friendly, homely nature for children, there would be two double guest rooms with bathroom and lavatory for the use of families. In addition, there would be a quiet room for discussions with, and between, parents and relatives. Besides the main kitchen, there would be a small kitchen for use by families. There would be a sluice room. Staff facilities would include a large general office and a staff sitting/meeting room. The document stated that a small mortuary chapel would be provided. However, the feeling of the meeting was that, because the hospice would not be exclusively Christian, the term 'mortuary room' (rather than mortuary *chapel*) should be used.

By far the most significant sentence in this section of the draft document about the planned hospice (at least as far as Richard and I were concerned) was the one that read 'Accommodation will be provided for eight children'. The size of the planned hospice was what Richard and I felt most strongly about, not least because we felt its size, more than anything else, would determine the atmosphere and quality of care to be found there. Helen House was to be based on the care and support Frances had given Helen and us; we did not feel that Frances's care could be scaled up beyond a certain level without it losing its very special quality. Moreover, Richard and I did not want Helen House in any way to resemble a hospital or an institution; we wanted it to be as homely, as much like a family home, as possible. We felt that while, admittedly, not many families had eight children, you could just about imagine a large Victorian family of this size. Perhaps, by wishing to emulate the Victorian family model, we were unwittingly embracing one of the few good points about the Victorian values our political leaders were soon to urge us to return to! Be that as it may, Richard and I felt that eight beds (not all, obviously, occupied all of the time, any more than all the beds in a family

82

home necessarily are) was the maximum number that should be provided.

A lengthy discussion followed about the size of the hospice. The view was expressed that building a hospice for eight would not be 'cost-effective'. I argued very strongly that cost-effectiveness was not our main aim and the meeting finally agreed that, although eight beds would not be cost-effective, in the case of Helen House, where a family atmosphere was top priority, this should not be the primary consideration.

However, the debate did not end with the meeting. Over the ensuing weeks doubts were expressed in various quarters on the wisdom of building for only eight. I have to confess that we badgered Frances endlessly on this. Our, in part instinctive, feeling that Helen House should not be allowed to expand in the planning stage (or, indeed, thereafter) led us to telephone Frances frequently, urging her not to waver but to stand firm even against expert advice. Since Helen House was a 'first' who were the 'experts' here anyway? I am happy to say that the quality-of-care argument won the day and Helen House has eight children's bedrooms. I cannot resist slipping in a word of advice, or rather the expression of a firm belief, at this point. You should never lower your aims for any reason whatsoever, whether of convenience, economy or ease. Since ideas are more often diluted than strengthened on the path to realization, you should, if anything, raise your sights beyond what you might realistically hope to achieve.

Having discussed the buildings and facilities the planned hospice should have, the meeting then turned its attention to the subject of costs and money-raising. The draft document stated that until detailed plans were drawn up, it would not be possible to make a precise estimate of the capital cost of the buildings, furnishings and equipment for the hospice. However, it seemed likely at that stage that the total capital costs would be in the region of £300,000. The running costs for a hospice of this nature were likely to be high since a high ratio of staff to children would be necessary. They were expected to be between £80,000 and £100,000 per year (in 1980 money values).

As soon as outline plans had been drawn up, money-raising for the capital cost of the hospice would begin. It was hoped that this sum could be raised through appeals to charitable and other organizations and from private donations. Appeals would also be made for covenanted subscriptions to contribute to the revenue costs. Discussions were currently taking place with the relevant authorities to establish the principle of financial support for individual children. No child would be excluded because of his or her family's inability to contribute financially. There would be no fees.

The draft document ended by saying that it was intended that a group of people to be known as the 'Friends of Helen House' should be established. This group would help with, among other things, the raising of funds locally. The hospice would come under the umbrella of the Society of All Saints in its status as a registered charity.

In the ensuing discussion it was felt that, since the raising of capital would almost certainly prove easier than the raising of revenue, every effort should be made to encourage support for the latter. It was felt, too, that the Charity Commissioners should be asked whether covenants made out to Helen House, without mention of the Society of All Saints, could still come under the umbrella of the Society in its status as a registered charity. In this way people would feel reassured that their contributions would be used only for the hospice. If this were not feasible, the possibility of registering Helen House as a charity in its own right would have to be explored.

The meeting ended with an agreement that 'Helen House – 12th May 1980' (the title of the draft document we had discussed at our meeting) would form the basis of an appeal leaflet, together with some information about the Society of All Saints, in whose grounds in Oxford the hospice was to be built.

The main action to be taken following our meeting on 16th May fell to the architect. It was agreed that John Bicknell would now start drawing outline plans and that he would approach the Planning Officer for the area informally to seek some assurance that there would be no major objection to the scheme in principle. In addition, Frances and I agreed to start working on the appeal leaflet.

Thus by May 1980 what had been simply an idea three months earlier was on the road to becoming reality.

5

The Vision Becomes Reality

A very purposeful atmosphere pervaded those early days of planning. The positive outcome in its own right was what everybody involved was interested in. There were no careers or reputations at stake or to be promoted. There were no professional or personal rivalries or jealousies. This was a great strength of the campaign.

Richard, Frances and I began work immediately on the appeal leaflet. This leaflet was prepared in our home. The three of us discussed the content and wording and Frances and Richard then drafted it while I took little Catherine out in her pushchair for forays to the nearby riverbank or playground. My input was thus punctuated by delightful excursions into the outside world with our second little daughter while Richard and Frances remained in charge of Helen – the inspiration and focus of our planning – as they wrote the leaflet.

The leaflet outlined the background to the planned hospice and gave the basic facts and information about it, clearly and simply. I feel we were lucky that at that time there was not the emphasis on slick and glossy promotion that we are told people expect nowadays even from charities. Of course we wanted to explain to potential supporters and users of the hospice we were planning what we had in mind but we were confident that those ideas themselves, simply put forward and explained, would be sufficient to make people wish to help. We would have found it difficult, and indeed inappropriate, to go for the hard sell we are told now lies at the heart of giving. This does not mean we were not then, or are not now, concerned with efficiency, effective management and success in the generating of funds and support, but simply that we do not believe that the only path to these is paved with glitz and gloss!

An expert in marketing and 'media manipulation' wrote recently of the dangers of 'unfashionable' charities missing out if they do not market themselves aggressively. Naive as this may sound to marketing moguls, I would suggest that by putting across the ideas behind the charity clearly and simply and with a minimum of 'packaging', you help to ensure that a charity does not become 'unfashionable' in the first place. After all, it is surely the style (both of the language and the packaging) that dates more than the underlying idea; it is their clothes and external trappings that go out of fashion more than the people within those clothes. Simplicity has much to recommend it, not only in terms of honesty but of *enduring* life.

Interestingly, when in 1980 the newly-appointed administrator of Helen House showed our recently-completed leaflet to a friend at the Institute of Public Relations, the latter confessed to being very impressed by the 'professionalism of its simplicity'! To the question he had asked the administrator before he saw the leaflet – 'What is your house style?' – the answer should perhaps have been: 'Simplicity and clarity.'

Because we realized the importance of establishing our credibility both in professional circles and generally, Frances approached a number of senior doctors in the Oxford area (including Helen's surgeon) and asked if they would lend their names to the Helen House project. This they were happy to do and their names appeared inside the front cover of our first full leaflet and on the front of the shorter version used more specifically for fund-raising purposes. Also on the front of the leaflet was a child's drawing of a house with a garden and a single blue forget-me-not. The tiny blue spring flower had been adopted as the emblem of Helen House; this was the idea of a friend, Clive Offley, who is a graphic designer and who was responsible for the layout of the leaflet and for the small, black and white photographs in the longer version. The drawing of the house (which in many people's eyes is almost as much a

symbol of Helen House as is the forget-me-not) is a drawing
that Frances herself did when she was five years old to send
to her brother who was very ill in hospital. By coincidence,
Frances's mother came across it when she was tidying out some
drawers in her home about the time we were looking for a
suitable drawing for the leaflet. Frances's childhood drawing
draws together very neatly several different very relevant
strands – children, Frances, home and illness. Above all, it
has proved to be an invaluable symbol of Helen House – a
house of homely dimensions which tries to be what *children*
themselves see as a happy welcoming home-from-home.

Fund-raising for Helen House began in 1980. It took the
form as much of exposing an idea as of asking for money. Of
course, by exposing the idea we hoped to encourage people
to support the hospice but we were anxious that the idea, not
the money, should be up front, that people should understand
the need for Helen House. This did seem to work; the idea
behind Helen House, once explained, seemed to generate
money. Our faith in the project also helped interestingly
enough, and to our amusement, it helped, in a sense, both
positively and negatively. There were those who identified with
our belief in the importance of the project and our confidence
that it would succeed and who therefore supported us
enthusiastically. Equally there were some who thought we were
hugely over-ambitious and unrealistic and that our project was
doomed to failure and who supported us out of pity. The only
way in which we asked directly for money was by writing to
the organizations listed in a directory of distributors of funds
for charitable purposes. Elsewhere the approach was to spread
the word and to put faith in people's understanding, empathy
and goodwill. Perhaps these are too often discounted.

We did, of course, in outlining our plans, need to tell people
how much we needed to raise to realize these plans. It was
now calculated that we needed £400,000 to build Helen House
and the annual running costs (measured in 1980 values) were
estimated at £100,000 because of the high ratio of staff to sick

children. However, in early press and radio coverage the emphasis was very much on putting across what was, after all, a rather novel idea. Helen House, when built, would be the first purpose-built children's hospice in the world. (The first broadly similar place, the children's hospice at St Mary's Hospital for Children, Bayside, New York, which was at a fairly advanced stage of planning when Helen House was first being discussed, did not in fact open until five years after Helen House, in 1987. Moreover, it is a 'hospice unit', alongside, and attached to, an existing hospital.)

The local Oxford newspapers printed their first articles about the proposed hospice in the summer of 1980. These articles bore a number of different headlines: 'Child inspires plan for care of chronically ill'; 'Nuns launch appeal for hospice cash'; 'Nuns plan city refuge for sick children'; 'Hospice inspired by Helen's suffering'. At the beginning of August 1980 Frances made her first broadcast about Helen House on BBC Radio Oxford. On Bank Holiday Monday at the end of August Frances and I were interviewed on Radio Oxford together and we described why Helen House was needed and what it would provide for very ill children and their families. Frances spoke of her gratitude to local people; between those two local radio broadcasts in August 1980, £5,000 had been donated to Helen House.

The first national media coverage of Helen House came in September 1980. An article entitled 'Going to stay at Helen's House' was printed on the Women's Page of *The Guardian* and immediately brought Helen House welcome supporters from all over the country. Even this national coverage (which in turn generated further nationwide media coverage) had a personal source and originated with Helen herself. While Helen was in hospital I had struck up a friendship with the mother of a young girl who for a short time occupied the bed opposite Helen's on the children's ward. This person turned out to be Prue Leith, then cookery writer on *The Guardian* newspaper. We remained friends after she and her daughter (completely cured of the problem that had occasioned her stay in hospital) left the Radcliffe Infirmary. When, later, we were planning Helen House she took a keen interest in our plans and was responsible for alerting the editor of *The Guardian* Women's Page (then Liz Forgan) to the project and the story behind it. The origin of this very useful article is another example of how many of the major decisions and the milestones on Helen House's journey from idea to reality were firmly bedded in some way in Helen's life.

From the moment the first articles about Helen House appeared in the press and the first broadcasts went out on local radio, money started to come in. An item in the *Oxford Star* of 9th October 1980, headed 'Hundreds help Helen Appeal', reported that the Helen House appeal had 'raised an incredible £76,500 in just eight weeks'. There seemed to be a great number of people who identified with the cause, or who wanted to help in some way. Inevitably, some of the keenest and most eager of the early supporters were personal friends either of Frances or ourselves. One of the first people to make a donation to our funds was the lock-keeper from Abingdon Lock; he loved Helen dearly and therefore regarded himself as very obviously a friend of the hospice that was to bear her name. People supported Helen House for all sorts of reasons. Many of the early supporters were keen to support it because it was a local initiative. Many people said it was 'something they could understand'. Families who had perhaps lost a child or who had friends who had been bereaved in this way identified with the families who might use the hospice. A large number of people empathized perhaps because they derived such joy from their own, or friends', well children that they had some inkling of what it must be like if a child close to you was afflicted with an incurable illness. A recurrent theme in letters from well-wishers and supporters was (and still is) their immense gratitude for the good health enjoyed by the children dear to them. Some people quite simply wanted to help what they felt was a worthwhile cause.

The excitement of those early days of planning and fund-raising is hard to describe or to recapture. A steady and gradually increasing stream of letters and donations came in day by day and added to our elation. We rang Frances, or she rang us, almost daily and she frequently came to see us bearing bundles of letters held together with paperclips which we pored over together. The size of the donations people sent varied enormously but we valued them all equally. What cheered us so much then was the growing *number* of our supporters; the success of Helen House would, after all, depend on an enduring understanding of what it was about and who it could help.

It was with this in mind that Frances travelled far and wide, talking to schools and clubs and small groups of all sorts about Helen House. She was soon a familiar sight in her habit, travelling the highways and byways of Oxfordshire and beyond with a large Paddington Bear, much loved by the primary school children she addressed, in tow! In the early days she travelled around in the estate car belonging to All Saints Convent (ever generous in their support) but later she was even more easily identifiable as she went about in a white Volkswagen Beetle belonging to the administrator of Helen House which he had had painted with the words 'HELEN HOUSE, a hospice for children, OXFORD' and a few forget-me-nots. The comment was made that all Frances needed was to have a large slit made in the top of the car to make it into a travelling collecting box!

In those early days Frances's most common ports of call were schools. A large number of schools adopted Helen House as their 'charity of the term' and were enthusiastic and ingenious in their fund-raising efforts on its behalf. Some schools held sales of their harvest produce in the autumn and of hand-made Christmas decorations and sweets in December, in aid of Helen House. Many gave the proceeds of school concerts, shows and bazaars to the cause. All sorts of raffles and games ('Guess the number of sweets in the jar'; 'Guess the score in the next school hockey match', etc.) were organized and children far and wide were sponsored to do anything from walking round their school field twenty times to keeping absolutely still for half an hour; from singing hymns non-stop to remaining silent for the entire lunch hour. School children wore their own clothes to school and then paid a fine for not wearing school uniform, the fine going into their collecting boxes for Helen House. Teachers (perhaps encouraged by the blissful silence in their school lunch hour!) joined in the fund-raising too, and in several schools the staff organized sponsored slims which left them fitter and better able to control their charges once the halcyon days of sponsored silences and purposeful walks were over!

The fact that so many school children felt so positive about Helen House and were so keen to help was immensely cheering and seemed very appropriate, too. Shortly before Helen House opened, Wheatley Park School near Oxford gave £3,500 to the cause. The Deputy Head of the school said that the children at the school had been incredibly enthusiastic about raising money for Helen House and that the sum they had raised in less than a year was the largest amount the school had ever raised for a charity in an academic year.

What was particularly gratifying was the young people's thirst for information, not only about what they could most usefully do to help, but also about the philosophy behind Helen House, and how the hospice would actually work. Frances spoke at assemblies and during general studies courses at schools up and down the county and beyond. She was indefatigable and impressed people wherever she went by her energy, enthusiasm, warmth, understanding and compassion. She found her visits to schools very interesting; I often think she would be well qualified to produce a guide to our schools and the atmosphere pervading them! She found her audiences in schools receptive and full of often disarmingly direct questions. Letters school children wrote to her after her visit show, by their directness and informality, how well the children related to Frances and her 'message' and how keen they were to contribute both money and ideas:

Dear Mother Frances,
 How is Helen?
We are sending some money for her house.
Love from Mary Rose.

Dear Mother Frances,
 Thank you for coming to my school to give a talk about Helen House. It made me realize how lucky I was to be a normal child with nothing wrong with me. To be honest I thought your talk was going to be very boring but write (sic) from the beginning it was really interesting.
 Please come again when Helen House is complete.

Dear Mother Frances,
 I have saved my pocket money for Helen House. Please send my love to Helen.
 Lots of love, Rosamond.

Dear Mother Frances,
 We are saving pennies for you in a bottle. I think you would need a settee and some towels.
 Love from Clive.

In the fund-raising for Helen House goodwill, enthusiasm, imagination and a sense of fun abounded. Our fund-raising predated the established, regular, much publicized efforts of Children in Need, Comic Relief, the Telethon Appeal and the like, and Helen House seemed to attract, locally at least, all the verve and energy which were later to be pumped in to these bigger, national ventures. The fund-raising itself generated a great sense of camaraderie and friendships were forged as people came together with a common aim. It was clear that many people feel a great need to get involved, to identify with a cause. Perhaps this is a symptom of an increasingly mobile and fragmented society where people feel more isolated and find it harder to satisfy their need to belong to identifiable groups.

Whatever their motives, hundreds of people threw themselves into fund-raising with zeal and were generous with both their time and money. The range of activities people organized to raise money for Helen House was enormous and we were amazed by some of the peculiar things people were prepared to do for a good cause! One local man was sponsored to shave off half his beard and to live with half a beard for a month. A trainee chef spent forty-eight hours sitting in a bath full of cold spaghetti in a well-known local hotel. Oxford Ski Club arranged for a former Olympic skier for England to 'ride' on roller skate skis from Oxford City Centre to Exeter Hall, Kidlington, a distance of six miles. The sisters of All Saints, Margaret Street, London joined forces with their congregation and with staff from John Lewis plc to do a five-mile tiddly-wink relay race in Oxford Street, London. As the headline in the *Marylebone Mercury* put it 'a wink is as good as a nod for fund-raising'. Three local motor mechanics organized a 'boat race with a difference', a sponsored dash across the River Cherwell and back on precarious, home-made rafts. There seemed to be an inexhaustible fund of ideas of ways to raise money!

What was gratifying about the fund-raising was that businesses and organizations of all sorts, as well as individuals, wished to contribute. Because of the wide cross-section of people and organizations who chose to support Helen House, donations ranged from the extremely large to the very small. I well remember Frances's excitement on receiving, at a fairly early stage in the fund-raising, a cheque for £75,000 from a charitable foundation. The cheque was accompanied by a letter politely requesting her to note that the sum enclosed was a one-off donation and did not constitute an annual subscription! At the other end of the spectrum, I remember how touched Frances was when a child who had filled a Smarties tube with pennies arrived at All Saints Convent to present the tube to her. One man turned up every Saturday to donate ten pence from his pension, from the moment Helen House was first mooted until he died a year ago. It is because of a generous gift of £40,000 from R.A.F. Brize Norton that Helen House has a jacuzzi.

Frances continued her extensive travels, talking about Helen House and, increasingly often, receiving cheques in all sorts of (sometimes improbable) venues. (I well remember accompanying her to a disco at a power-station where she was plied with Blue Nun wine!) How she maintained the energy and enthusiasm which made her words unfailingly inspiring in their freshness and conviction is something we can only wonder at. The blurb in the *Radio Times* advertising a radio documentary programme about Helen House which was broadcast in the week the hospice opened, was not far from the truth when it said that Frances 'made the average movie nun look rather dozy'! (And nobody would suggest that Maria in *The Sound of Music* lacked energy!)

There were other figures who played a key role in the foundation of Helen House but whose contribution is only fully recognized, perhaps, by those closely involved with the hospice. One such person was Sister Benedicta. She was a member of the community and somebody who loved Frances dearly and recognized her special talents and gifts very early on in their association. Her role in the birth of Helen House was a crucial one. First and foremost, it was she who identified Frances as the right person to be nominated for the position of Mother Superior General when the previous incumbent's period of office came to an end in 1977. I think it is fair to say that had Frances not been Reverend Mother at All Saints Convent when we met her shortly after Helen was taken ill in 1978, Helen House would never have come into existence. Frances's vision, faith and stamina, her personal attributes, her love of children and her insight into the needs of sick children, combined with her authority as Reverend Mother and the respect in which she was held in that role, were of fundamental importance in ensuring that Helen House, metaphorically and literally, got off the ground.

Sister Benedicta was a catalyst in the development of Helen House in other ways too. She was responsible for recruiting two key figures on the Helen House staff – the Administrator, Michael Garside, and the Head Nurse, Edith Anthem. Sister Benedicta joined the community comparatively late in life. She did not become a nun until she was forty-five. Before that she had had a full and varied professional and private life, working as, among other things, a literary agent. Her interests were wide and it was through her work as Honorary Organizing Secretary for the Wildfowl Trust in London in the late 1950s that she got to know Michael Garside, who was then Personal Assistant to Peter Scott at the Wildfowl Trust in Slimbridge. Sister Benedicta (or Ray Gregorson as she then was) effectively vanished from professional life for seven years and it was only years later, when she came to visit Peter Scott and his family, wearing a black habit and a wimple, that Mike understood her reasons for withdrawing from public life. Even though Sister Benedicta obviously no longer worked for the Wildfowl Trust in any capacity, she remained a friend of Peter Scott and his family and a regular visitor to their Slimbridge home.

It was on a visit to the Scotts in July 1980 that Benedicta was responsible for changing the direction of Mike Garside's life and thereby doing much to ensure the smooth running of Helen House. Mike went to meet her at the station to drive her to the Scotts' home. In her characteristically forthright and direct manner, Benedicta told Mike that the sisters at All Saints Convent were trying to raise one and a half million pounds. Mike's response was that the sisters were mad; there was no money around. He asked what on earth the project that required such funds might be, to which Benedicta's answer was that it was a children's hospice.

Nothing more was said then, but Benedicta left a copy of the recently prepared proofs for our leaflet on the seat of Mike's car. He recounts how, when he read the leaflet, he was deeply

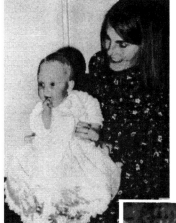

Helen, aged four months, on the day of her christening, 25th April 1976.

Below: Helen, just six weeks before her brain tumour was discovered, en route to the compost heap with some vegetable peelings.

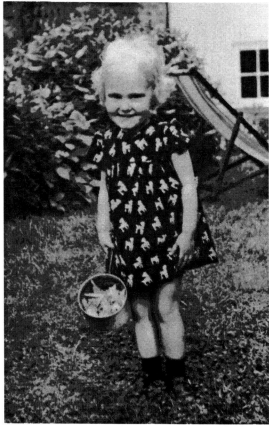

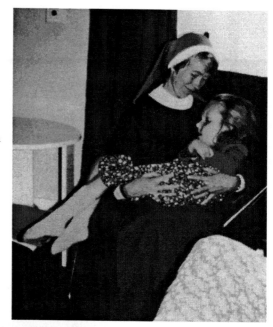

Helen with Frances
on one of her short
stays in Frances's room
at the convent.

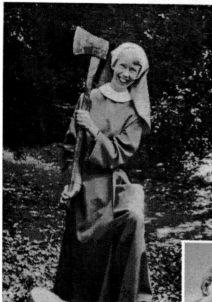

Mother Frances lends a hand
when the builders first move in
to clear the site for Helen
House, summer 1981.
(Oxford & County Newspapers)

Below: The model of Helen
House made by members of
the Architects Drawing Office
at Harwell in their spare time.
(AEA Technology)

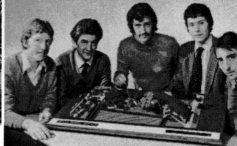

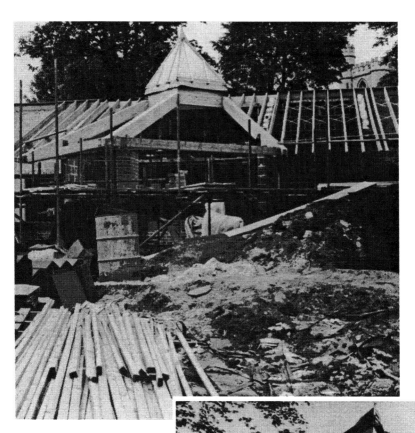

Building work under way.
The imaginative triangular
design created a building of
intimate proportions and
architectural interest. In
1983 the building won the
highest award given by the
Oxford Preservation Trust.

(Julia Baker)

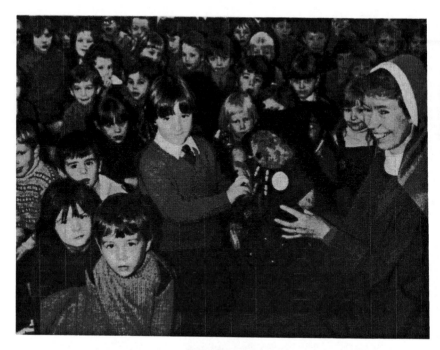

Mother Frances on one
of her many visits to
schools. Here a pupil at
Dunmore Infants School,
Abingdon slips a cheque
for Helen House into
Paddington Bear's pocket.

(Oxford & County Newspapers)

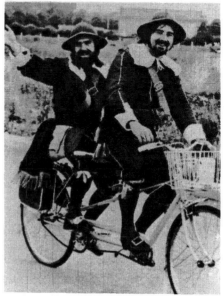

Right: Two members of
the Sealed Knot Society
cycled 105 miles to the battle field, stopping along
the way to collect money
for Helen House.

(Oxford & County Newspapers)

Right: Firemen from RAF Brize Norton completed a sponsored walk from the air base to Helen House wearing breathing apparatus.
(RAF Brize Norton)

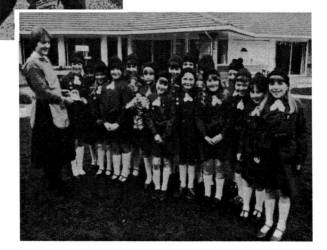

Left: A 'guess-the-weight' competition organised by a local butcher swelled the funds.
(Oxford & County Newspapers)

Below: Pip Leitch, deputy head nurse, receives a cheque from a local Brownie pack.
(Oxford & County Newspapers)

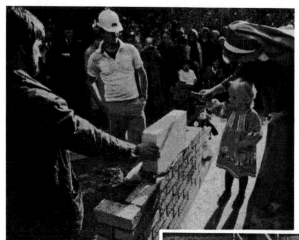

Helen's sister, Catherine, lays the foundation stone – with a little help from Mother Frances Dominica – 27th October 1981. *(Oxford & County Newspapers)*

Right: The topping-out ceremony, August 1982. John Bicknell, the architect of Helen House, is second from right. *(Oxford & County Newspapers)*

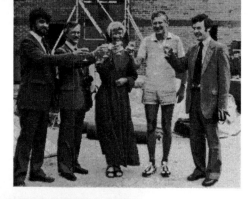

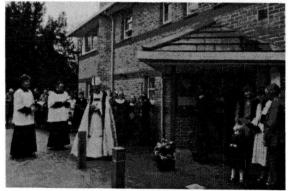

The Blessing of the completed building by The Bishop of Oxford, Patrick Rodger, 4th November 1982. *(Oxford & County Newspapers)*

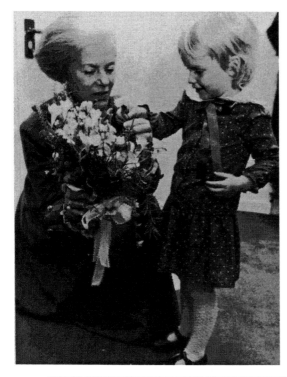

Helen's sister, Catherine, chooses a flower from the bouquet she has just presented to HRH The Duchess of Kent at the official opening, 30th November 1982. *(Oxford & County Newspapers)*

Below: The front of Helen House from Leopold Street. Above the entrance hall and office is the parents' accommodation. *(Nigel R. Barklie)*

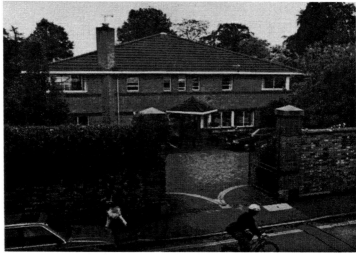

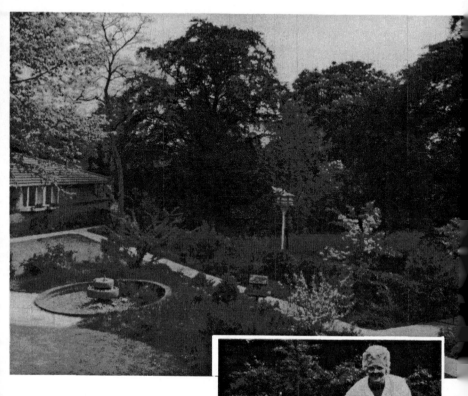

The view from the balcony of the parents' flat across the Helen House garden to the convent garden beyond.
(Nigel R. Barklie)

Right: Edith Anthem, head nurse, enjoys a walk around the garden with Colin.
(Nigel R. Barklie)

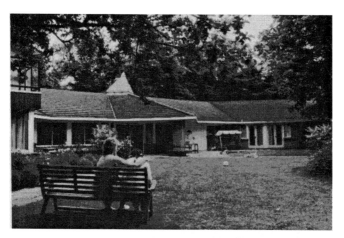

Above: Samantha enjoys a peaceful moment in the garden with Doreen, one of the team. In summer the garden is often the scene of picnics and barbecues. *(Nigel R. Barklie)*

Right: Kate feeding her daughter, Natalie, in one of the bedrooms. *(Nigel R. Barklie)*

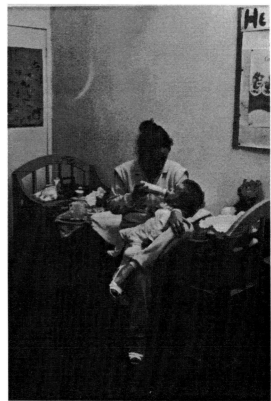

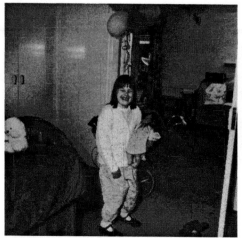

Becky in a characteristically happy mood. The inter-connecting double doors between some bedrooms can be kept open where children wish to share.
(Nigel R. Barklie)

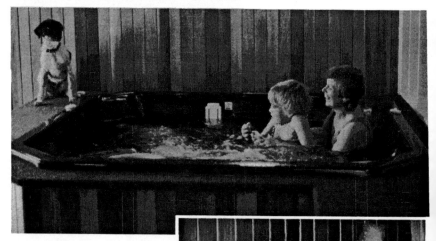

The jacuzzi, a gift from RAF Brize Norton, provides endless enjoyment.

Above: Jamie takes a dip with Vron, a member of the team, while Tish looks on. *(Nick Foden)*
Right: Wayne smothers Kenny, a member of the team, with foam. *(Nigel R. Barklie)*

A special ballet lesson
for Susan from a member
of the Sadler's Wells
Royal Ballet, who visited
Helen House as part of a
touring project.
(Oxford & County Newspapers)

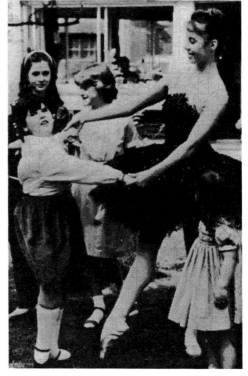

Below: Helen and Stephen
cuddle their daughter,
Victoria, during a stay at
Helen House.

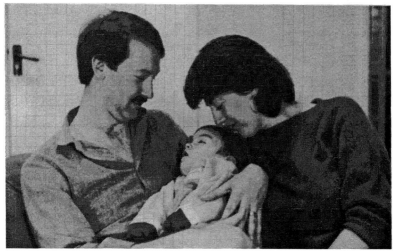

A very important member of
the team - Tish. A recruit from
a local animal sancutary, Tish
now lives with the Deputy
Head, Eve Herd, and comes
into the hospice when Eve is
on duty. *(Nick Fogden)*

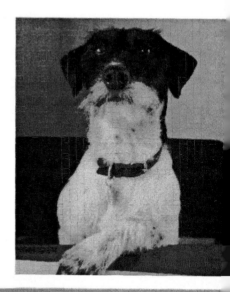

Below: The playroom is the
focal point of Helen House.
The main building is all on one
level and access to the garden
is easy for Craig and other
wheelchair users. *(Nigel R. Barklie)*

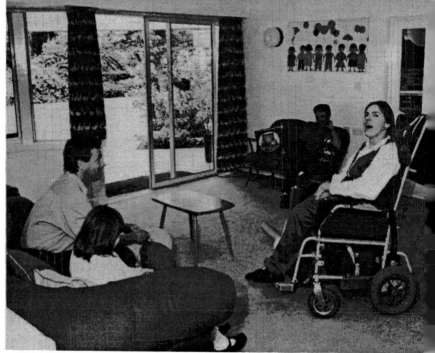

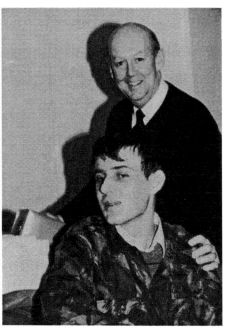

Mike Garside, the administrator, with Douglas who, like his sister Penny, came regularly for respite care at Helen House.

Below: Matthew enjoys a cuddle in the playroom with footballer Glen Hoddle.
(Oxford & County Newspapers)

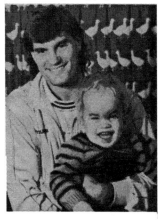

Bottom: Brothers Ian and Wayne in the garden. *(Nigel R. Barklie)*

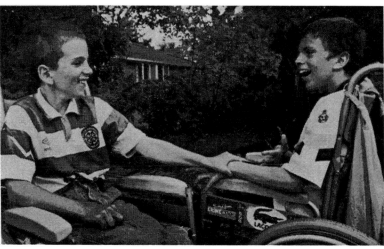

Right: Leanne.

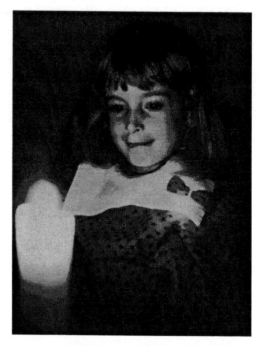

On the hospice's
fourth birthday Mother
Frances received the
Templeton UK Project
Award from financier
John M Templeton
(right). Richard, Isobel
and Catherine blow
out the candles on the
birthday cake.
(Oxford & County Newspapers)

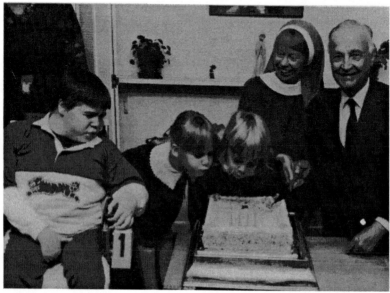

Helen House

When you get to Helen House.

You go to which ever room you go to.

The one I'm in at the moment is Willow.

And then you can go through the door.

And on the wall is Hellow Susan in fancy writing.

There is 8 bedrooms all together 2 toylets. and two baths.

But there is jacuzzi

You put water up to the top. and there is two buttons one which shooters come into your back. and the other which bubbles on top.

There is a room with hundreds of books all diffrent orthers.

Also lots of story tapes and song tapes

We have a video and we can have any vidiow you want.

You have a tv and a tape recorder which you can have have. songs and storys.

When the children are bord you can sew you can draw play games moke things.

If you wont to you can have breakfast in bed

Also you might have a bit of choclat cake for tea.

There is these beem bags

If you really go there you will you would like it

It is like a hotel

Susan Peterson

After Susan wrote this at school, her school friends asked when *they* could come and stay at Helen House!

Ten years on, schools still take a keen interest in Helen House. Catherine, Helen House secretary, receives a tenth birthday gift from pupils of Great Haseley primary school.
(Oxford & County Newspapersr)

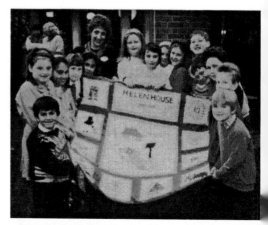

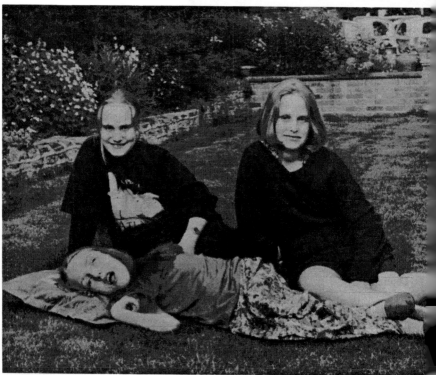

Helen, Catherine *(right)* and Isobel – three sisters together at home, June 1993. *(Nigel R. Barklie)*

moved and impressed and on the Sunday afternoon when he drove Sister Benedicta back to the station he told her that if there was any way in which he could help the Helen House project she should let him know. The sort of involvement he had in mind was perhaps running a small fund-raising group in Gloucestershire. Sister Benedicta had other ideas. She asked Mike if he would come and run the Helen House office. When he agreed, she told him that in that case it was *he* who was mad, not the sisters, because he was leaping from a secure position of twenty-five years' standing into the unknown. However, she did nothing to dissuade him!

Sister Benedicta reported back to Frances who followed up Sister Benedicta's conversation with Mike with an immediate interview with him (Frances had previously met Mike but the acquaintance was slight) to confirm arrangements. Having been identified and recruited by Benedicta in July, Mike arrived to take up his post running the fund-raising and administrative office for Helen House on 27th October 1980. He was the first member of staff appointed.

It was Sister Benedicta who decided that the hospice inspired by Helen should be called Helen House. This was obviously something agreed on early on, as headings to the minutes of early meetings make clear. What Benedicta also proposed was that Catherine should lay the foundation stone of the hospice which was to bear her sister's name. This was an inspired decision and a poignant reminder of what Helen House would do and how it had come about. Catherine represented not just her sister Helen, the inspiration behind Helen House, but children generally and of course Helen House was to help children. She also represented the family of a sick child and Helen House would aim to provide support for families too. Above all she was full of life and invested with so many hopes, and our fervent hope was that Helen House would provide the best possible quality of life for the ill children who visited it.

Even after Sister Benedicta herself became ill (she was diagnosed as having cancer in 1982) she continued her active role in the 'shaping' of Helen House. While she was staying in the Churchill Hospital she was nursed by someone who impressed her greatly. The more she got to know this person, the more certain she was that she had both the personal qualities and the professional skills to make her ideally suited to overseeing the day-to-day running of Helen House. Edith Anthem (who was to become Head Nurse of Helen House) recalls how Benedicta one day asked her, out of the blue: 'Why aren't you nursing children?' Benedicta told Edith about Helen House and arranged for her to meet Frances and ourselves in addition to Roger Burne and Mike Garside. Edith took up her position as Head Nurse on 20th September 1982, just under two months before the first children came to stay.

Sister Benedicta, who died in September 1983, was a catalyst in the development of Helen House. It was a project very dear to her heart. When she was told that she had cancer, she declared herself 'fed up' because she might not be around to see Helen House actually up and running. She announced her determination 'to be around for the opening' and in fact she lived for ten months after that date.

The loss of Sister Benedicta was keenly felt, not only by the sisters of All Saints, but by everybody involved in the setting up of Helen House. For Frances the loss was probably greater than for anyone else. In Benedicta she had had a loving, supportive and wise friend, endowed with great compassion and, above all, common sense. Moreover, Benedicta was as forthright in her criticism as in her praise. She had a knack of identifying the root of a problem and was able to extract what was of lasting significance from the surrounding, often redundant, detail.

The arrival of Mike Garside, Sister Benedicta's first recruit to the Helen House staff and, indeed, the first paid member of staff, made an immediate impact, as I am sure Benedicta knew it would. Mike was to run the office, at that time based in the guest wing of the convent, from which fund-raising, publicity, planning and administrative matters relating to Helen

House would be co-ordinated and managed. Everything relating to Mike's appointment and arrival in Oxford fell into place with uncanny ease. One striking example of this relates to his salary. A charitable trust to whom Frances had written to appeal for funds for the hospice had written back to say that, while contributing to building costs was outside their terms of reference, they might be able to fund a salary for two or three years. Frances wrote back immediately to say that as it happened, although Helen House was not yet operational (or even built!), she was about to make the first appointment to its staff in the form of an Administrator. Perhaps the foundation would like to pay his (modest) salary for two years? This they were happy to do and thus for the two years that Mike worked for Helen House before it opened, overseeing the planning, building and fund-raising, his invaluable work imposed no financial burden whatsoever on Helen House.

Mike's arrival in Oxford coincided with a sudden upsurge both of interest in, and fund-raising for, Helen House as people came to hear about the hospice by word of mouth, through press and radio coverage and through Frances's talks. It would have been difficult for those working in the office in the convent guest wing to continue to cope unaided with the ever-increasing number of letters and donations that this growing interest and awareness inevitably generated. Mike's arrival on the scene was timely. He immediately installed the usual charitable accounting system – the roundabout accountancy system with cash book, bank records and 'flimsies' (individual records of every donation made). He set about getting to know everybody and everything related to the Helen House project and soon had all the relevant information at his fingertips. He kept (and still keeps) scrupulous records of all Helen House business, meetings and appointments and of fund-raising activities, correspondence and enquiries about the hospice or visits from potential helpers or from interested professionals. He was soon the key figure in all discussions with the architect who designed Helen House and it was soon to Mike that everybody went for Helen House information. His role gradually evolved into what it is today. Broadly speaking, it involves everything that is not nursing care; Mike is in charge of administration, finances, investments, salaries, maintenance of the Helen House building and the establishment. In addition, like other members of the staff of the hospice, he goes out all over the place giving talks about Helen House and receiving donations on behalf of the hospice. However, although his role as Administrator is what distinguishes him in most people's eyes, he is known to many families as much more than that. His real understanding of what Helen House is about and his empathy with the children and families who come to the hospice have meant that some of those families have looked to Mike for more than (excellent) advice in practical matters; for them he is a friend.

Mike's success as Administrator of Helen House stems from his attitude to his job and his character. His calm, courteous and direct approach to people and his readiness to tackle a problem at source have made him extremely effective in his professional role. He confronts problems without ever being confrontational. Economy could be his watch-word. He does not like to see energy (and I am referring to light bulbs here, as well as physical exertion!) wasted. His ruthless honesty can be disconcerting at times; he will say what he believes is right even if it is not what you might wish to hear. He would never compromise his principles. Thus, in his eyes, the frugal approach he always favoured in the early days of fund-raising, when we had no idea how hugely generous people would turn out to be, has not become any less appropriate now, simply because Helen House has attracted large sums of money. In fact, Mike would probably argue that our duty to be frugal is clearer than ever; the greater people's generosity, the greater our responsibility to use their gifts carefully and effectively.

Mike is rigorously fair and this can be uncomfortable at times. He has proved uniquely able to safeguard the principles underlying the running of Helen House, when in all the success surrounding the hospice it might have been easy to lose sight of those principles. Sister Benedicta's wisdom in appointing him is apparent to us all.

One of the first people with whom Mike Garside had dealings when he came to Helen House in the autumn of 1980 was the architect who designed the hospice, John Bicknell of Bicknell and Hamilton in London. John Bicknell was not unknown to the Society of All Saints; he had designed the Novitiate and Guest House and the Bethlehem Chapel in the grounds of All Saints Convent. He was keenly interested in the idea of Helen House and attended all the early meetings of the group initially involved in the discussion and planning of the project. As agreed at the end of our meeting in May 1980, John Bicknell went away to draw outline plans for the proposed hospice and to approach the Planning Officer for the area to seek assurance that there would be no major objection to the scheme in principle.

By July 1980 he had completed outline plans and these were discussed at a meeting on 11th July 1980. The meeting expressed enthusiastic general approval of the plans which were then discussed in detail. The minutes of the meeting show how the discussion was underpinned by a general recognition of the fact that Helen House should seek to mirror a family home not a hospital or institution and by the desire to do everything possible to enhance the homely atmosphere in the place, even though clearly at Helen House there would be features and provision that no ordinary family home would encompass. This is clear from points in the discussions about the mortuary and about the seminar room. Regarding the former, it was felt the mortuary should be a single-purpose room and should be designed to look as much like an ordinary room as possible, perhaps even with ordinary windows. It would certainly not be a cold, tiled room with no natural light. There should be a refrigerated bed against one of the walls and the room would be furnished like a simple sitting room.

In the event, the mortuary room is even more like a small

sitting room than we originally envisaged. It is furnished like a room in a family home. There is no refrigerated bed; a domestic cooler keeps the temperature very low when the room is serving as a mortuary room. Between times the room can be used by anyone seeking a comfortable, intimate place for reflection or quiet conversation. It also houses a wooden cabinet containing the book of remembrance in which the names of Helen House children who have died are beautifully inscribed.

As regards the seminar room, the fact that groups would be likely to visit the hospice and would need a room in which to meet, hear talks and perhaps see films was discussed. The general opinion was that it would be a pity to alter the character of Helen House by including a sufficiently large seminar room for such meetings and gatherings. It was agreed that it would be preferable to use other accommodation, possibly in one of the convent buildings.

Although the personal/human dimension was ever-present in our minds we were, of course, not blind to important medical and nursing considerations. Though Helen House would be as much like a family home as possible, it would incorporate features that would ease the problems both of the ill children themselves and of those nursing them. For example, it was felt that in the children's bedrooms a basin with 'push handle' taps, easily accessible to a child in a wheelchair, was preferable to a basin in a vanity unit. The inclusion in the plans of wheelchair toilets is another obvious example.

The attitude to the possible provision of a hydrotherapy pool further illustrates the approach of those who attended the early planning meetings. At the meeting in July 1980 the architect was asked to make provision, in his more detailed plans, for a hydrotherapy pool, though we realized that in the event we might not raise enough money for this facility to be included. While we were full of hope and optimism, these feelings were tempered by frugality, by the realization that we should not set out to be lavish; our responsibility was to seek to provide the basic facilities combined with the right staff and atmosphere, rather than to aim, before we had even gauged the public response to our plans, to provide luxury accommodation of the five-star hotel variety. At a subsequent meeting in November 1980 (which the architect said would probably be the last meeting necessary to examine architect's drawings; he envisaged that tenders would be let in April 1981) the feeling was expressed that the subject of the hydrotherapy pool would need to be discussed further in detail. If it did prove possible, because of the generosity of the public, to provide such a facility, it was felt that the current proposal for a stainless steel unit was too expensive and, significantly, too 'clinical'.

At this stage there was no detailed discussion of what is a much-appreciated feature of Helen House today – the garden. I think we all took it for granted that Helen House would have a beautiful garden. The therapeutic value of gardens (and gardening) for people suffering from stress is now widely recognized. Beauty and contact with natural rhythms and with the pace of nature (rather than with the nerve-fraying and unnaturally frenetic pace of many of our lives) can bring great peace, acceptance and a relaxation of tension. The children who would come to stay at Helen House might not be able to look forward to a long life but every effort would be made to ensure that the quality of whatever life they still had ahead of them would be as high as possible. To be able to run and play (if they were strong enough) in beautiful, natural surroundings, to be wheeled in their wheelchairs, or to sit or lie, in the fresh air, amidst trees, shrubs and flowers, listening to birdsong and smelling the scent of earth, grass and plants would, we felt, contribute enormously to this quality of life. Richard and I remember vividly how, during Helen's long stay in hospital, we longed to whisk her away from the clinical smells and 'manufactured noises' of the ward and give her a taste of the natural world. One afternoon in that beautiful Indian summer of 1978 we carried her down to an inner courtyard in the hospital where there was a small area of grass.

Though she was still deeply unconscious at this stage, her rigid little limbs relaxed visibly in the gentle warmth of the sun and in the fresh air.

In his final plans, John Bicknell specified in quite precise detail how the Helen House garden should be landscaped. Evergreen shrubs of different heights would give interest (and year-round 'clothing') to a low central mound area which would also include a small pond. Here a fountain would splash over stones, providing a soothing sound but never filling the pool and thereby making it a hazard. There would be a beech hedge masking the very necessary wire-mesh fence between the Helen House garden and the convent garden. The plans allowed for a couple of existing trees to be protected and to be incorporated into the final lay-out.

Richard and I have always been involved in the Helen House garden. In the early days of planning we were keenly interested in its design both because of our interest in gardening and because we believe that the importance of beauty is too often underestimated in the process of healing (in its broadest sense) and in therapy. Moreover, we felt that if, when Helen House opened, we had no occasion to use the hospice facilities as such (we had no idea how long Helen might live) to be involved in planning, digging, planting and pruning in the garden would mean we had a very obvious reason to simply be around quite frequently. I am sure we needed to feel that we would have an active and continuing role in the development of (to quote many young supporters) 'Helen's House'. To watch over and foster happy, healthy growth, while this can be poignant when contrasted with the impaired development, and indeed the withering, of young lives, is very sustaining and comforting.

A further meeting of the 'committed group' (referred to, often, now as the Helen House working group) was held at the end of September 1980. At this meeting there was further discussion of points of detail and John Bicknell submitted his target programme. One matter that was discussed on this occasion was the question of a possible model. The opinion of the architects was that to have a scale model of the proposed building would be too expensive. The feeling of the meeting was that, though a model would be nice, it was an unnecessary expense. Richard intervened here. He felt that a model would be invaluable in helping us all to get a picture of what the hospice we were busy planning would really look like. Anyone who has had any building work done on their home or an extension built (or who has studied planning applications at the local council offices) will know how difficult it is to get a real feel of the end product from architect's drawings and from elevations on paper. Richard felt that with a project as important as this we needed to be absolutely certain that what was planned was right. I think that Richard and I were further motivated by a desire to ensure that the building that would bear Helen's name would, if you like, be worthy of her. Richard asked for agreement that he should try to arrange through contacts at work for a scale model to be made; this agreement was forthcoming. The next day Richard approached the head of the architect's department at the Harwell Laboratory and it was agreed that if Richard provided all the necessary materials the apprentice architects would generously give of their free time to build a scale model of Helen House from John Bicknell's drawings.

While this model was being built, John Bicknell was understandably anxious when asked to hold fire and not to produce further detailed drawings or indeed to incur any further costs relating to the existing plans until, on the information provided by the model now under construction, these plans had been cleared. However, we felt we had to be sure and that future confidence and certainty would compensate for any passing inconvenience or embarrassment at this stage.

On 15th January 1981 Frances and Mike Garside visited Harwell to see the completed model built by the apprentice architects. Like Richard, when they saw the model they were worried. Like him, they did not feel the planned building was right. It was altogether too imposing; it was not sufficiently intimate in style. It was agreed that it would be necessary to ask John Bicknell to make substantial modifications to his existing plans.

The delicate task of approaching the architect and explaining our misgivings about his plans fell to Mike. John Bicknell listened carefully to the points Mike made and then disappeared and came up with a new set of plans with remarkable speed and adaptability. These plans were felt to be much more promising but to be really sure Richard again approached the apprentice architects at Harwell and arranged, on the same conditions as before, for them to make a scale model from the plans. This they did and the finished product caused great jubilation. Not only was it a work of art in itself, but it showed a building much more like what we had envisaged Helen House would be like. We now felt, after the temporary lull in activity imposed by the 'model episode', ready to proceed at full steam.

The model itself helped enormously with fund-raising and with spreading the word and raising public awareness of the Helen House project. Over the next couple of years it was displayed in a number of prominent places, in banks and in the windows of High Street building societies, to name but two. It attracted a lot of attention because of the attention the Harwell apprentices had themselves given to detail, to bringing out the human dimensions of the hospice, to making it look in some way alive. One amusing story relates to the figures to be seen in the building and in the garden of the model. Because Helen House was to be built in the grounds of All Saints Convent and because Mother Frances was, so to speak, its figurehead, the people who constructed the model thought, in common with many others in those early days and, indeed, a good number of people still today, that the hospice would be staffed exclusively by nuns. Scale figures of nuns were not readily available for architect's models but, because of the boom in construction projects in the Middle East at that time, scale models of Arabs were. The resourceful apprentices bought a job-lot of mini Arabs and simply painted their flowing robes

106

to look like nuns' habits! It is said that behind every great man there is a woman; in this case behind every nun was an Arab!

In a sense then, Helen House as we see it today is Helen House mark two. The working drawings for the hospice which today welcomes sick children and their families from all over Great Britain are dated April 1981 and are the ones that John Bicknell prepared in response to our concerns about the original plans. An interesting detail at this point is that in April 1981 when those plans were finalized, the sum in the Helen House bank account stood at £233,000.

The fact that John Bicknell chose to act as site manager for the building project simplified things considerably. When the plans went out to tender he handled the proceedings. A press release issued jointly by the Helen House Administrator, Mike Garside, and R. Fuller, Director, Messrs. Newcombe and Beard Limited with the title 'Oxford firm wins Helen House contract' followed a meeting between John Bicknell and the building firm Newcombe and Beard on 14th July 1981 when the contract for the project was signed. Work was to start not later than 24th August 1981 and the contract was for a period of fifty-two weeks. The press release further stated that Mother Frances Dominica and the Sisters of the Society of All Saints had been overwhelmed by the generosity of hundreds of people throughout Britain and abroad who had given over £370,000 to the project since it was launched in August 1980. Additionally they had received £75,000 with which to set up an endowment fund. Excitement was the order of the day.

It is perhaps helpful at this point to give a summary of a few key dates. These show how relatively quickly things took shape.

February 1980	The idea emerged
March 1980	First informal meeting to discuss idea
1st September 1980	Outline planning permission obtained

107

A House Called Helen

7th January 1981   Full planning permission granted

August 1981   Building work started

and (jumping forward)

November 1982   Helen House opened

When Helen House opened the building was paid for.

The press coverage of the impending start of the Helen House building programme led to intensified activity in the fund-raising field. Cheques and donations to funds arrived daily and people continued to come up with novel ideas for raising money. As regards the building work, this began with immense enthusiasm and a sense of purpose and commitment. Some readers may be familiar with the book *I Leap Over the Wall*, the autobiography of a nun who felt unable fully to embrace the religious life and in this book describes her dramatic departure from convent life. Nobody leapt over any walls at All Saints Convent but a very significant moment in the birth of Helen House came when the Reverend Mother Frances Dominica allowed the wall of her convent garden to be broken through by a bulldozer. The day the bulldozer broke through the wall is generally regarded as a significant turning point, the moment when plans and ideas started to take concrete form.

The building work proceeded smoothly and efficiently. The site foreman on the Helen House project (who now has his own business and has regular dealings with Helen House, doing maintenance and repair jobs for the hospice) has spoken of the enthusiasm of all involved in the building work, of their interest in the project. The well-worn jokes about builders and time schedules would certainly not be appropriate here.

Fund-raising for Helen House continued apace. The hospice seemed to have a universal appeal – universal both in the sense that it appealed to all sorts of people and in the sense that interest in it was certainly not confined to the locality in which it was being built but stretched even beyond England. Service personnel on ships in the Falklands during the Falklands War collected money for Helen House and Helen House was the charity of the year for the R.A.F. in 1982.

The wide appeal of the Helen House cause was the subject of a leader in the *Oxford Times* of August 1981, entitled 'And now the good news':

'It is cheering in these troubled times to hear this week of the outstanding success of the Helen House Hospice in Oxford. It is an appeal that has touched the hearts of thousands of people not only in the Oxford area but in other parts of the country. In twelve months a staggering £417,000 – more than £1,000 a day – has poured in, raised by young and old at a variety of events, great and small. By any standards the response to the appeal has been phenomenal.'

The following year a leader in another local paper spoke of the 'remarkable campaign' to raise money for a children's hospice and called it 'an astonishing feat of organization and charity':

'All manner of people have been involved, not least the ordinary men and women of the city. Policemen and children, firemen and Welsh exiles, Rotarians and weight-watchers, insurance men . . . everywhere the heart has given gladly.'

The highlight of 1981 for us was the laying of the foundation stone of Helen House on 27th October. As Sister Benedicta had suggested, this was performed by Helen's two-year-old sister, Catherine, 'helped' (as the words on the foundation stone, now set into the wall next to the main entrance to Helen House, put it!) by Mother Frances Dominica. The week leading up to the occasion took its toll of the furniture in our home. We had explained to Catherine that on the day she would have to tap a stone with a sort of hammer and say some traditional words: 'This stone is well and truly laid.' She was unflagging in her efforts to perfect her performance of this ritual; for a week before the great day she went round our house with a wooden spoon practising on any solid piece of furniture that came to hand!

A House Called Helen

October 27th was a glorious autumn day. The air was crisp, the sun shone and the trees in the convent garden were beautiful in their autumn colours against a brilliant blue sky. The good weather meant that Helen in her wheelchair and our third daughter Isobel, now eight months old, could be present, which was what we had so much hoped would be possible.

We could not know what Helen might be absorbing from the occasion but our youngest daughter, Isobel, whose reflective nature coupled with an at-times-barely-contained and humorous zest for life have brought us great joy from the day she was born, made her appreciation of the morning's events quite plain; though she remained very quiet as she sat in her pushchair next to Helen, she beamed and kicked her legs throughout.

A good number of people had gathered to witness the laying of the foundation stone; friends, well-wishers and supporters, building site workers, sisters from All Saints and residents from St John's Home, a small group of young people with disabilities from Ritchie Russell House, members of Frances's family and of our family, Helen's surgeon, Mr Briggs, Roger Burne and his wife – the faces of these and many others can be seen on the film made of the occasion by Independent Television. There was a tremendous feeling of happiness and hope in the air. The laying of the foundation stone was also a very poignant occasion for Richard and me. The cruel curtailment of Helen's physically and mentally active 'well' life had, after all, led to this occasion and when the concrete and enduring reality of Helen House started to be apparent to us, the enduring, fixed and irrevocable nature of Helen's condition hit us afresh. The contrast between Catherine, brimming with life and good health, and the children who would come and stay at Helen House was also, inevitably, present in our minds. As we looked at the solid foundations of the hospice we could not help reflecting on how frail are the foundations of so many hopes and plans.

Catherine smiled and had a look of quiet contentment on her face throughout the performance of her important task, for which she was given a special mallet with a brass plate on it with details of the occasion and the date, which I am sure she will show to her grandchildren in years to come. Frances steered her gently through the ceremony, which was probably more daunting to Catherine than her calm, smiling appearance suggested, for, when asked by Frances, after she had tapped the stone and said her words, if she would like to do it again, Catherine's answer was a *very* firm 'no'! The TV cameras and press photographers were perhaps a little unnerving; her efforts with a wooden spoon in our home had, after all, escaped such public attention!

Frances and Richard both made short, informal speeches after Catherine had finished with the mallet. Frances was clearly deeply moved by the occasion; to see the product of her vision and her unflagging efforts in support of that vision begin to take solid form must have been quite overwhelming. As she stood next to the foundation stone (on which were carved the words 'Laid by Catherine, aged two, sister of Helen, helped by Mother Frances Dominica. 27 October 1981') she spoke briefly of her joy and of her immense gratitude to all who had helped bring us to this historic day. Richard was very happy to have the chance, for the first time, to thank Frances publicly for all that she had done for us and to underline that Helen House had arisen from the close friendship between Frances and Helen and ourselves. Friendship was, in a sense, the foundation stone of Helen House. Richard outlined to those present how Frances had on several occasions had Helen to stay with her in her room in the convent where she had looked after her with great love and gentleness and he said that Helen House would be quite simply 'Frances's room at the convent eight times over – and, of course, thanks to the amazing generosity of so many people, it'll have one or two other facilities as well!' If ever a project had a clear remit it is Helen House.

The other very significant 'pre-opening' event in the Helen House calendar of 1981 to 1982 was the blessing of Helen

House by the Bishop of Oxford, Patrick Rodger, almost exactly a year later. As we stood amidst the mud and bricks on the building site on 27th October 1981 we would have found it hard to picture ourselves a year later, on 4th November 1982, standing outside the completed Helen House, a warm, welcoming and beautifully furnished building. The blessing of Helen House was a very joyful occasion, particularly, I think, for the sisters of the Society of All Saints, who saw in Helen House both the fruits of their prayers and hopes and an immense opportunity for future (and growing) Christian and pastoral work in the wider community. In a short ceremony, the Bishop asked for God's blessing on Helen House. With his chaplain beside him and preceded by a thurifer and a sister with holy water and accompanied by a small group of representative members of the assembly he went all around the building, asperging and censing the rooms and offering appropriate prayers at each point. In one of his final prayers, he prayed that all who ministered at Helen House and all those they cared for should find fullness of life and know the serenity of God's love and joy and peace.

It was a very moving occasion and one which served to remind us that Helen House would be a place where love would abound, where the wider issues raised by serious illness, impairment and death would be ever in our minds, a place where the *whole* child would be cared for and where the spiritual dimension would never be overlooked.

An important task during 1981 to 1982 was that of deciding on, and then purchasing or having made, the necessary furniture, fixtures and fittings for Helen House. Several meetings of interested parties were held to discuss the basic furniture that each room should have but most of the actual choice of styles, materials and fabrics fell to Frances and myself and I have to say we thoroughly enjoyed the task. For me, this creative activity was a welcome antidote to some of the time-consuming and sometimes fruitless struggles Richard and I continued to have with the various bodies responsible, to procure for Helen the basic provision (allowances, wheelchair, home support and aids) to which she was entitled. Frances often recalls how we constantly referred to Helen as we chose patterns and fabrics; 'Would Helen approve?' is a phrase that still often passes our lips.

In our choice of furniture, carpets, curtains and linen we were guided all the time by the wish to make Helen House as homely and friendly as possible. Because it would not be in any way an institution, Helen House would not have uniform furnishings in all the bedrooms; each bedroom would be decorated and furnished in a different style. This was important, too, if we were to cater for different tastes, for different ages of children and for boys as well as girls. The rooms would not be numbered but for the purpose of easy reference would be distinguished by names. The eight bedrooms each bear the name of a tree: Oak, Ash, Beech, Willow, Lime, Sycamore, Mulberry and Chestnut. An overriding concern was that everything at Helen House should be warm and bright, but not *aggressively* so; to avoid the cold and clinical you do not have to go to garish extremes! In this context, I once spoke to a wheelchair supplier who said his instructions were to cover all wheelchairs for children in bright orange material, to 'make them cheerful'. However, you cannot, as simply as his instructions might suggest, catapult people with disabilities or illness into cheerfulness; moreover, the very *violence* of the attempt would be off-putting to many!

In addition, Frances and I, and all who were involved, bore in mind the importance of considerations such as easy care and maintenance. We were also ever-mindful of medical and nursing considerations. The beds provide an interesting illustration of the marrying of what could be seen to be mutually exclusive aims – the desire to make Helen House as much like a family home as possible and the wish to ensure that the needs of the staff working at Helen House were borne in mind as they would be in a hospital environment. We realized that for the sake of staff lifting children in and out

113

of bed or perhaps bending over the bed to give them blanket baths it was important that the beds should be the height of a hospital bed. At the same time we wanted the beds to look homely and wanted them to be made of wood; not only are metal-framed hospital beds rather stark in appearance but Richard, Frances and I vividly remembered the distress caused to Helen in hospital by the loud clanking of bed sides being raised and lowered on the ward. This is why the beds at Helen House are specially-designed, purpose-built beds, made of beautiful ash wood but the height of standard hospital beds.

The large circular table in the dining area of the kitchen is another example of the marrying of very different considerations. It is a beautiful wooden table on a central stand and both its size and its design are important. The table is large enough to seat a very large family – in this case any children who might be staying and who are well enough to sit up to the table for a meal, members of their families and those looking after them on that particular shift. Moreover, the design of the table means it is accessible and can be used by people in wheelchairs. In addition, of course, its circular shape creates a very friendly atmosphere, one in which everyone feels included and as closely part of things as anybody else.

The wooden furniture in Helen House was manufactured locally. One day Frances came to see us at home in Abingdon. The annual craft fair was on at the time, in the Abbey Buildings just down the road from our house. One of the exhibitors at the craft fair that year was a local firm that makes wooden furniture. At a friend's suggestion, Frances and I went to look at the furniture and studied the wood from which it was made. We felt that furniture made of ash would look beautiful at Helen House and it was at the Abingdon craft fair (which Helen had previously enjoyed) that we first enquired about the purpose-built beds in the children's rooms. The same firm (then called Crowdys Wood Products, Clanfield) made bedside units for the children's bedrooms, the dining chairs to go with the circular table and all the furniture for the parents' flat. They have added further items down the years, all in the same wood, such as the waist-high gate between the dining area and the kitchen area which is invaluable when, for safety reasons, it is necessary to restrict access to the cooking area. Recently they made the wooden cabinet which houses the Book of Remembrance.

We were aware that we must always bear in mind the cost of what we chose in the way of furnishings and buy carefully to avoid waste (for example of fabrics). We must never be careless (or carefree) in our spending of what was, after all, other people's money. We were immensely fortunate, though, in that a lot of people volunteered to meet the cost of particular items, and shops and businesses too were generous with discounts. Ironically, though, it is frugality of approach at Helen House that has led in some instances to lavishness of provision. I think that because the administration of Helen House was seen to be mindful of expense and essentially frugal in approach, people felt moved to offer us a number of luxury items we could not have justified buying ourselves. Mike Garside tells the story of how in the very early days of fund-raising he used to avoid wasting paper by using the backs of the letters people had written and sent with their donations as the paper on which to write his notes of thanks. This led to one man writing to send a further donation because, he said, he had been impressed by Helen House's refreshingly unusual approach to cost-cutting! Further evidence, too, that not everybody responds to the glossy approach to fund-raising.

There were a considerable number of people at this stage who wanted to give not only their money but also their time and talents. We obviously wanted to tap all potential sources of help and also (and this we felt to be very important) keep those who had helped in any way informed of what was going on, of how their donations and efforts had benefited the cause. An important figure in this context in co-ordinating things was Heather de Freitas. She worked for the Health Authority, as

115

co-ordinator of the nurse bank, and had come forward at an early stage in the planning of Helen House to offer her services. It was she who set up The Friends of Helen House and who was responsible for establishing the tradition of the regular Helen House newsletter. The first newsletter was sent out to supporters in January 1981 and a second followed in the September of that year. The early newsletters were written by Heather de Freitas and kept supporters up to date with progress on the building front and with fund-raising and gave them information about events in aid of Helen House which they might wish to attend or support. The newsletter was invaluable, not only in establishing (and now, I believe, maintaining) a network of supporters, but also in enabling people to understand what Helen House is about and how their contribution (whether of time or of money) had been used and in making them feel that their efforts were appreciated, as they most certainly were. Heather de Freitas also organized the first Helen House sales of Christmas cards and notelets and, in the early days, of items which are no longer available such as ties, headscarves, tea towels, badges and lapel pins. Christmas card sales and all-year-round sales of cards and notelets are still an important source of revenue.

The inevitable and growing media interest in Helen House was not without problems for us in the early days and indeed has been difficult for us on occasions since then. Helen House was a 'first' and therefore bound to attract considerable interest. Although all of us concerned were at pains to stress that Helen House was to fill a gap in existing provision, that it did not seek to replace any service already available or indeed wish to imply by its existence any criticism of any service currently available to sick children and their parents, Helen House was nevertheless seen in some circles as controversial and controversy fuels public interest. One very senior local paediatrician declared himself unable to see why Helen House was needed. As he explained, if a child was very ill he could not believe he or she would not be accommodated in hospital.

116

If the parents were managing to look after the child at home, what was the problem? (We have come a long way since then.)

Moreover, the story of how our beautiful, bright, lively little Helen had been transformed into a totally helpless little individual was the stuff of which many a highly-coloured, emotionally-charged tabloid newspaper story of the human interest variety is made. The fact that Helen House was designed to help gravely ill children was the final lure and made it an obvious source of material for those wishing to balance their emotionally arid news items with something designed (to quote one) to 'tug at the heart strings'. Articles and items about Helen House in the press were peppered with words such as 'plight', 'agony', 'tragic', 'plucky'; one local free newspaper trots out the phrase 'tragic kiddies' in almost any, even passing, reference to Helen House! The fact that Helen House was inspired by the serious illness of a dearly-loved small child, that it was a world first, that it was founded by a dynamic (and very photogenic!) nun and that later Royalty was involved gave it irresistible appeal for the media.

Our position in all this was a difficult one. We wanted above all to protect Helen and our family generally from any intrusive publicity. We felt that to expose little Helen's total helplessness to public view − particularly when, as is very often the case especially with television coverage, the exposure is in the context of public entertainment − was, at best, unnecessary and, at worst, inexcusable. Helen, after all, was not in a position to say no or simply to run away from the cameras! We felt that, although Helen had obviously inspired Helen House, the idea behind the hospice and how it would operate could be put across to the public quite adequately and indeed very well without attention being focused voyeuristically on Helen herself. Perhaps the intelligence and imagination of the general public are too often underestimated or, indeed, set at nought.

Nevertheless we did from time to time − usually at moments of stress or passing discouragement − re-examine our feelings on these matters because of course we were aware that public awareness of the needs of families with very ill children had to be heightened if Helen House was to attract support and be a success. However, we always returned to a feeling of certainty that publicity for the cause need not entail sacrificing peace and privacy for Helen. The delicate balance between privacy for an individual and the need for publicity for a cause that has perhaps come to the fore because of something that has occurred in the life of that individual is one that it is hard to maintain.

In an attempt to shield Helen from the glare of publicity, whenever I spoke on the radio about Helen House I asked to be referred to simply as Helen's mother, because we have a rather distinctive surname and I did not wish to be tracked down at home. Similarly, in press articles about Helen House or press interviews we did not use our surname. On occasions this had amusing consequences. In local newspaper articles covering the very happy occasion of the laying of the foundation stone of Helen House in October 1981 comments by Richard about the occasion were prefaced by such remarks as 'the girl's father, who did not wish to be named, said . . .'. Our desire for privacy made us appear on occasions slightly shady!

We were, of course, prepared to provide all the information about Helen and ourselves necessary to an understanding of how Helen House had arisen and why it was needed, but not to offer Helen up on the media altar. Our instinctive wariness of the media proved to be well-founded, as one particular incident demonstrates. This incident which, as well as being distressing for us, helped to foster misunderstandings which still persist, occurred on what should have been a day of unclouded happiness for everybody concerned with Helen House, the day of the blessing of the building by the Bishop of Oxford on 4th November 1982. Although Helen was ill on the day, we had felt she should be present in the building when 'her' house was blessed before it opened its doors to the first children two weeks later. We took her to one of the Helen

House bedrooms and made her comfortable in her wheelchair. She was very sleepy and because she was quite unwell – she had chickenpox quite badly – she looked extremely pale. We had been warned that a television journalist had expressed an urgent desire to get pictures of Helen and the blessing but since we had explained that Helen was very unwell and had made it clear that in any case it was not our policy to expose her to cameras, we thought no more of it.

Our shock on seeing the lunch-time news on ITV that day was immense. Not only was a picture of a desperately ill-looking, pale and very still little Helen blazoned across the screen – it had been taken from behind bushes in the convent garden with the aid of a telephoto lens trained on the bedroom in Helen House where Helen was dozing in her wheelchair – but the accompanying 'news' text was inaccurate in a very distressing way. Its strong implication was that Helen did not live at home with her family, but was now resident in Helen House which had been built by Mother Frances for children like Helen who needed somewhere to live when they became very ill (and therefore unwanted by their families?). The implication was that, far from loving and caring for her at home, we had abandoned Helen on her becoming ill. As the 'news' report put it: 'Helen's hope lay in Mother Frances.' Not only was this news item upsetting for us, but of course it did Helen House a disservice by suggesting that Helen House was a place that offered long-term residential care, not a place that would offer continuing friendship and support to families with very sick children and on-going, short-term, respite care for those children.

Mike Garside was quick to react. Through the solicitor who acted for the Society of All Saints, he took out an injunction. The tasteless, distressing and inaccurate news item did not appear on later ITV bulletins that day. Perhaps journalists like the one who crept around the convent garden with his telephoto lens, showing precision in the use of that tool of his trade but a disregard for truth worthy of the legendary Matilda, never stop to consider the pain their insensitivity and the false information they disseminate causes those whom they so blithely misrepresent and on whose feelings they trample.

One problem which perhaps we might have avoided if we had allowed more publicity for Helen herself or indeed courted publicity ourselves rather than chosen to be active from the wings so to speak rather than on the stage, is that many people think that Helen is dead, indeed has been dead for many years. They believe that Helen House was inspired by her but now stands in her memory. This, coupled with the other common misunderstanding, namely that Helen lives at Helen House and only comes home to us for special occasions like Christmas and birthdays or for short holidays, seems very difficult to eradicate.

Although we are wary of television and of media coverage generally, we fully recognize that there is good and bad in television as in everything else. Early in 1982, a half-hour documentary programme about the foundation of Helen House appeared on ITV. It was a programme in the *Jaywalking* series, presented by Sue Jay. It began with a biography of Frances and an explanation of how she had come to embrace the religious life. It described briefly the work of the religious community of which Frances was Reverend Mother and moved on to describe how Frances's life and work (and that of the community, too) had taken on a new dimension following her meeting with Helen and with us. The programme told Helen's and our story briefly and outlined how Helen House had come about and how it was hoped it would operate when it opened. The programme ended on a note of great hope, with the laying of the foundation stone of Helen House.

The success of this programme lay in its being thoroughly and conscientiously researched and in the presenter, Sue Jay, and the other researchers being prepared to listen to those they talked to and respond to what they heard and adapt their own views where necessary. Admittedly, to begin with Sue had struggles with those above her who favoured a much more sensational approach and to whom restraint and understatement were clearly dirty words. We received letters from Sue's bosses and a visit to discuss possible filming of Helen and ourselves at home and once again there was a danger that the 'tragic kiddies syndrome' might go into overdrive. However, long and careful discussion between those involved and Frances and ourselves led to significant changes in attitude and approach and the end product was something we were, broadly speaking, very pleased with. What helped enormously was that Frances and I were allowed to go up to Birmingham to see the completed film to check that we were happy with it and to make minor changes where necessary. The programme that finally appeared on the screen produced an enormous and appreciative response and was variously described as very moving, interesting, informative, inspiring and sensitive. One of the producers did actually get in touch afterwards to say that the treatment of the subject and the approach we had insisted upon had proved to be 'absolutely right'. We felt vindicated in our unswerving belief that to capture people's interest and, indeed, to move them, you do not need to go for the emotional jugular with quite the brash gusto that is sometimes exhibited in such cases.

Once the building was complete and furnished, all that remained to be done before Helen House welcomed its first children was to give the public a chance to see what they had helped to create. It was, after all, the generosity of hundreds of individuals as well as the support of companies, organizations and charitable institutions, which had made Helen House a reality. It was felt that those individuals who wished to do so should have the chance to come in and see what Helen House was like, to see where the children with whom they had so clearly empathized would sleep and eat and spend their waking hours when they came to stay. So it was that the series of open days was held. For three days in November 1982 Helen House was open house to a constant stream of visitors whose interest and delight in the building, the furnishings, the facilities and the toys were very encouraging. On those open days the queue of people waiting their turn to enter Helen House stretched down Leopold Street and round the corner into the Cowley Road. There was certainly no public awareness problem here!

With Helen House the informal has, in a sense, nearly always displaced the formal. The pattern was set right at the outset; the formal, official opening of the hospice by H.R.H. the Duchess of Kent took place on 30th November 1982, a fortnight after the first two children to come and stay at Helen House had been warmly and informally welcomed.

Most of the people who take an interest in Helen House are aware that its patron is H.R.H. the Duchess of Kent and that it was she who officially opened the building in November 1982. What they are probably not aware of is how it was that she came to be involved in Helen House and the amount of discussion that took place relating to the merits (or otherwise) of patronage and the wisdom of involving famous people in a venture whose hallmark was to be privacy and informality. All sorts of different views were expressed on the subject. It was felt by some that there was really no need for any famous person to open Helen House, nor indeed for Helen House to have a patron. On the other hand, having a patron, particularly if it were somebody who was held in high public esteem, known and respected, would give Helen House a credibility which it could perhaps otherwise lack. We were only too aware of the problems some people might have in believing that Helen House could establish itself successfully and function professionally, indeed even go from strength to strength, based as it was on something 'non-professional', the friendship between a nun and a very ill small child and her parents. Judgements made on the basis of future possibility rather than on the basis of past fact require a certain faith, independence of thought and an open-mindedness which are not always forthcoming. Perhaps, then, it would help to strengthen Helen House's professional credentials and avoid it being seen as the touching, but possibly unsustainable, whim of a benevolent nun and a 'distraught mother' (to quote one tabloid!) if it had a high-profile patron?

When we discussed who the patron of Helen House might be and who might open it, there were all sorts of considerations to be borne in mind. It was important that we should avoid bolstering, by our choice of patron, any false impressions of Helen House and its aims. One such impression was that Helen House was run by a religious community exclusively for the children of families of the same faith. For this reason, to have a Church of England dignitary to open it would be unwise, in that it would serve to strengthen that impression. Helen House was intended to help any family and their sick child, irrespective of faith, colour, creed or background. Just as it should not, therefore, be associated with any one particular faith, so, equally, it should not be associated with any one political party or with a person of any particular and stated political persuasion. To have a minister or politician open it would be wrong. (I have to say we never found this option at all tempting!) Helen House was intended to last, to have an enduring life. For this reason it would be unfortunate for it to be associated with an 'ephemeral' character, with a popular, but perhaps passing, star. In any case, because it was to be a place of support, refuge, tranquillity and privacy for ill children and their families, association with someone who obviously courted publicity was inappropriate. Clearly anybody who could be seen as in any way controversial was to be avoided.

The discussion continued. Because of Helen's (and his own) love of music and our and Frances's belief in the therapeutic power of music and in its ability to nourish the spirit even (or especially) where the mind and body are perhaps impaired, Richard felt that it would be appropriate for a musician to open Helen House and be its patron. However, we were aware that Helen House was to cater for all and not everybody has the same taste in music and we wanted at all costs to avoid the

123

accusation of exclusivity. Moreover, we really needed somebody we could feel confident that most people had heard of, somebody whose name would mean something to just about everybody, somebody who was, in a sense, 'public property'.

Our thoughts turned to the Royal Family and, at Frances's mother's suggestion, to one member of the Royal Family in particular, largely, I have to say, because of her Christian name – Lady Helen Windsor, the only daughter of Their Royal Highnesses The Duke and Duchess of Kent. Although of course members of the Royal Family are in one obvious sense members of a particular class – a very privileged and exclusive class at that – the Royal Family is in a very real (and somewhat baffling!) sense 'public property'; people from all walks of life consider the Royal Family to be just as much theirs as anybody else's.

We decided that Lady Helen Windsor should be approached to find out whether she would be willing and able to become Patron of Helen House and whether she would consider officially opening the hospice in the autumn of 1982. Having sought advice on the protocol, Frances wrote a letter in January 1981 to the Lady in Waiting to H.R.H. The Duchess of Kent asking if it might be possible to approach Lady Helen Windsor with an invitation to this effect. She enclosed the Helen House leaflet and expressed the belief that it would give the project enormous encouragement if H.R.H. The Duchess of Kent would allow her daughter to become involved. She further stressed that Helen House had no formal council and therefore held no meetings; its business was governed by the trustees of the Anglican Society of All Saints. This meant that Helen House would very rarely call upon Lady Helen's time.

The reply from York House was disappointing. The Lady in Waiting to H.R.H. The Duchess of Kent thanked Frances for her enquiry but said that she regretted it was not possible for Lady Helen to undertake any patronages or engagements at that time. She explained that it was the express wish of the

Duke and Duchess of Kent that none of their children become involved in any public engagements until they had all completed their education, which would not be for several years. Having thought about this, we decided that we would like to invite Lady Helen's mother, the Duchess of Kent, herself to perform the opening ceremony. By the end of June 1982 the invitation had been accepted and the choice of a mutually convenient date was all that remained.

It was the Duchess's own wish, expressed after her first visit when she officially opened the hospice, that led to her becoming its patron. I have to say that we could not have a more dedicated and involved patron. H.R.H. The Duchess of Kent is in frequent contact with Helen House and takes a great interest in everything that goes on there. Since she opened the hospice in 1982 she has visited it regularly. The children and families greatly appreciate her warm interest and she is dearly loved. The only problem for her in this context is, perhaps, what Gloria Steinem refers to as 'empathy sickness'; H.R.H. The Duchess of Kent feels acutely for all the sick children and their families that she meets. She is very much in tune with the aims of Helen House and the spirit of the place. She has, moreover, been delightfully affected by the infectious informality of Helen House and, improbable as it may sound, on her visits to Helen House informality certainly outweighs formality!

The first visit of H.R.H. The Duchess of Kent to Helen House, however, when she came to open it was obviously a somewhat more formal occasion. The Duchess arrived accompanied by a Lady in Waiting and by the Lord Lieutenant of the County, Sir Ashley Ponsonby and his wife, Lady Martha. In the entrance hall she unveiled a plaque (it bears the words 'This building was opened by H.R.H. The Duchess of Kent on the 30 November 1982.') and made a short speech. The first two words of her speech were 'Mother Frances' and the last word 'Helen'. Catherine (now aged three) presented Her Royal Highness with a bouquet of flowers and the Duchess then toured Helen House and met the eight ill children and their families in the hospice on that day.

Lunch was served in Helen House for all present on that momentous day. Among those seated around the friendly circular table in the kitchen/dining room were Her Royal Highness The Duchess of Kent and her Lady in Waiting, Frances, ourselves, John Bicknell and his wife, Sir Ashley and Lady Martha Ponsonby, the Lord Mayor (the Reverend Tony Williamson) and the Lady Mayoress and Major Henry Garnett (Chairman, Cancer Relief). On subsequent visits to Helen House by Her Royal Highness, lunch has become an increasingly informal affair and is now usually a buffet meal with everyone, adults and children alike, circulating freely.

The headline in the *Oxford Mail* that evening, above the article accompanying the photograph of Catherine and the Duchess read: 'Duchess opens happy hospice'. The Duchess herself speaks of being quite overwhelmed by Helen House. That she should have commented on the aspects that we felt were so important was immensely cheering to us. 'The feeling of happiness here is practically tangible – the atmosphere so warm and welcoming; the house vibrant with colour and sunshine.'

6

After the Opening

Helen House welcomed its first two children on 15th November 1982. In an interview on the *PM* programme on Radio 4 that day, Pip Leitch, the Deputy Head Nurse, spoke of the role of Helen House and told listeners a little about the first two children to come and stay there. They were a boy aged nearly two and a girl aged twelve. The boy and his family lived locally; the girl came from Anglesey. Thus at the outset a pattern was established which has not changed down the years; Helen House continues to welcome both boys and girls and these are a mixture of local children and of children whose families travel a considerable distance to bring them to the hospice.

There had been a huge build-up to the opening of Helen House; it was, therefore, perhaps inevitable that there should be a feeling almost of anticlimax when the hospice actually opened. Everybody involved in the planning and in the lead-up to the opening, giving talks to interested groups and organizations and spreading the word either formally or informally, had stressed the very important role Helen House would play and had talked about the great support it would give to gravely ill children and their families. When Helen House opened, this fine mission statement had to be translated into action. This was for real.

The first weeks and months in the life of Helen House were a period of adjustment. The staff needed to settle into their role, to gain confidence that what they were doing in practical and human terms really was what was enshrined in the powerful words that had been used to describe Helen House before it opened. It was perhaps inhibiting (as well as being a source of pride, which of course can in itself be inhibiting) that Helen House was a 'first', that so much had been said and written about it before it opened. The problem for staff was, I think, to connect all the little things they did day by day for the children temporarily in their care and for their families with the stated aims, purpose and philosophy of Helen House. Love, friendship and support are such dauntingly all-embracing words; but of course what they denote is compounded of a host of small, commonplace and oft-repeated actions. Some staff had real problems here, I feel; they needed reassurance that the numerous, seemingly trivial, little things they did for the children and families in their care were not a pale shadow or a dim reflection of the grand overall aims of Helen House; together they all contributed to the realization of those aims. Abstract concepts are nourished, sustained and given their meaning by a host of small practical deeds. In so many discussions about caring nowadays, this is forgotten.

Richard describes the atmosphere at Helen House in those very early days as like that of a new shop opening and awaiting its first customers. There was a definite tension and nervousness in the air. The staff really did want to test out on somebody the shop assistant's well-worn opening gambit: 'Can I help you?', without, of course, bearing down intimidatingly on those who might cross the threshold of Helen House and come and see what it had to offer. In the context of Helen House every word of that short sentence 'Can I help you?' would have real meaning. The staff would need to relate to each individual 'you'; each 'I' on the staff would need to test out his or her individual ability to help and that help might take all sorts of unexpected forms. However, fairly predictably, families did not come flocking to Helen House the moment it opened. Staff needed to remember that inevitably it would take time for Helen House to become really busy. It was, after all, a new and untried idea and the number of families to whom its services were relevant was, thankfully, limited, although larger than might generally be supposed. Furthermore, not all families with children who might be seen to fall within the description of 'Helen House children' would choose to use Helen House. This immediately distinguished Helen House from a casualty department or an acute hospital ward offering active medical treatment aimed at cure, to which almost every parent would clearly take their child if his or her illness or injury seemed to demand it.

In those early 'waiting days', then, patience and quiet confidence were what was needed in rich measure, but for staff keen to test their skills, these were hard to summon up. They were particularly elusive for the less self-assured and for those who had come to Helen House from a busy hospital background. There was an additional problem here, too, – that of guilt. A few of the staff spoke of feeling guilty at not having enough to do at Helen House in those early days as they waited for families to want to turn to them for help.

Another source of uneasiness at the outset stemmed from the sort of children Helen House had been set up to help and the way these children had often been described. The children would be children with a life-threatening illness, children for whom active treatment aimed at cure was, sadly, no longer appropriate. This had quickly become 'dying children' in much talk about Helen House and in most articles and features about the hospice. (To be fair, this was perhaps for reasons of brevity as much as for dramatic impact.) For some of the staff in those early days there was a feeling that until a Helen House child had actually died Helen House had not, in a sense, established its credentials. There was anxiety on a purely personal level too, which was perhaps greatest among those many staff members who had not got any sort of 'medical background'; how would the death of a child affect them? Some of them felt that until they knew this they could not gauge their suitability for the very important job they had undertaken to do at Helen House.

In those early waiting days, when there was more that was unknown than was known, one person remained stubbornly impervious to doubt or anxiety. This person was Edith

Anthem, the Head Nurse, who took up her post at Helen House in September 1982 just two months before the hospice opened. In those first weeks and months Edith kept a level head and a firm belief and confidence that it was only a matter of time before Helen House would be welcoming a large number of sick children and their families and before the unknown became the known. Indeed, it was all to the good that in this hitherto uncharted territory, staff should have the chance to find their way gradually, to adapt to the very varied demands of their role, to share experiences and feelings in an unhurried atmosphere and to establish a firm foothold in what was, inevitably, uncertain and even shifting terrain. Edith's quiet confidence that all was, and would be, well, was an invaluable fillip to staff morale.

Edith Anthem was identified as the right person for the job of Head Nurse of Helen House by Sister Benedicta who was nursed by Edith at the Churchill Hospital during the last weeks of her life. Edith grew up in Lancashire and she describes her childhood as happy and secure. Her younger sister, who was born when Edith was four, suffered badly from infantile eczema and Edith remembers the district nurse calling daily at their house to change the dressings on her sister's sores. Her sister was also prone to asthma and required much tender care. Edith recalls that at the age of four she felt that what she wanted to do in life was look after children but not to nurse them; she made a definite distinction there.

It was Edith's father who launched her on a nursing career when she left school by drawing her attention to an advertisement in the local paper for cadet nurses at Alder Hey Children's Hospital. Edith applied and was accepted as a cadet nurse. To her own surprise as much as anyone else's (her aunt had been very sceptical about Edith's ability to cope with the rigours of nursing life and had said that she would pay her ten shillings for every year she stuck at it!) Edith loved cadet nursing. She loved everything about it, including cleaning the lockers and all the mundane little jobs. Having spent three years at Alder

Hey Hospital she moved in 1955 to St Helens General Hospital, where she did her general training before returning to Alder Hey, where in 1956 she qualified as an S.R.N. and in 1957 as an R.S.C.N.

Having gone south to do a midwifery course at Queen Charlotte's Hospital in London, Edith was recalled to Lancashire by the illness of her mother. Throughout her childhood Edith had always been aware that her mother was not strong; she suffered badly from rheumatism and had a weak heart and Edith had always felt that her mother needed her care almost as much as she and her sister needed their mother's care. Even as a young child she had somehow instinctively known how to ease her mother's anxiety and discomfort and had found joy in so doing. It was perhaps not surprising that when, all those years later, her mother became more seriously ill it was to Edith that she looked for support and indeed that it was Edith who wished to nurse her.

Over the next four to five years Edith gained first-hand experience of the difficulties faced by families caring, day in day out, for a much-loved sick or disabled relative. On her return from London she spent six months nursing her mother at home. In 1959, when she married John, whom she had met two years previously whilst nursing at Alder Hey, the family brought someone into the home to care for her mother to enable Edith to set up home with her new husband and also devote more of her energies to the job she had recently taken on, that of Nursing Sister at Pilkingtons Glass Works in St Helens. However, Edith remained closely involved with her mother's care and became even more involved after February 1962 when her mother had a massive stroke while Edith was with her one day. Although Edith and her husband lived fifteen miles away from her parents' home and now had an eight-month-old baby, Edith's energy and devotion made it possible for her mother to be cared for at home and to be rehabilitated to a significant degree. For a time Edith had her mother living with her, an arrangement which only came to an end when the family GP 'put his foot down' a month before Edith and John's second son was born and insisted that nursing care should be arranged for Edith's mother in her own home.

Edith remembers vividly the circuitous and tiring bus journeys she made to visit her mother after work in the early days of her illness and again in the later stages, after her mother was once again in her own home. I think her own experience of the problems many people often face visiting relatives in hospital is further amplified by the first-hand knowledge she must have gained over those painful years when her mother was so ill. She has more than an inkling of the pain caused by conflicting loyalties and by (often unsuccessful) attempts to share energies and attention fairly, and the physical exhaustion and heavy undertow of sorrow which are the daily diet of so many of the families who come to Helen House.

After her mother's death in 1963 Edith's energies were largely devoted to her family and to voluntary work. When her second son was three years old, Edith started to do night work as a sister on the paediatric ward at the local hospital. Part-time nursing was to be a feature of her life over the next few years. This was possible because Edith had a close friend who was a health visitor and they took it in turns to look after each other's children. Edith later decided to do a Health Visitor's course herself but when she applied in Liverpool she was told to get some practice in the district. To this end she embarked on school nursing, which she did for two days a week. The school nurse in those days was concerned more with diagnosing the problem and treating it once it had arisen than with education aimed at preventing it arising in the first place. The emphasis was on the problem rather than on the individual children. Edith would have liked to have the chance to take a more holistic approach to the care of the children she met all too briefly on her whistle-stop tours of schools.

In January 1970 Edith's husband, John, was moved by the bank he worked for to Oxford. Edith describes her horror on learning that they were to move south. The south of England was alien territory to her. Her only incursion into this land she viewed with such suspicion had been when she had done Part One of her midwifery course in London before her marriage. She had disliked the course intensely and this had done nothing to enhance her view of the 'unfriendly' south. It was with a heavy heart that she upped sticks and moved to this area where she and her family have lived ever since.

On arriving in Oxford, Edith wrote to the Churchill Hospital envisaging doing perhaps two nights a week nursing. She realized she could not pursue her idea of doing a Health Visitor's course, because she no longer had the back-up of a close friend with whom to share child care, so she decided to try to do the next best thing and nurse children in hospital. However, when she was called for interview she was dismayed to learn that she would not be able to undertake paediatric nursing in her new home area because 'Oxford trained its own paediatric nurses'. She remembers feeling angry as well as bitterly disappointed. She agreed to go on the nursing bank, working initially one night a week but later, and for eleven years, for two nights a week on the gynaecological ward. Although at various times during that eleven years she was offered daytime work, she always declined because she did not want to leave her children. When it was suggested to Edith that she should apply for a night sister's post she again declined, but for a very different reason; as she explains it now, she did not want to walk around with a clipboard, she wanted to be involved with nursing. Edith was then, and is now, a 'hands-on' person. This does not mean she is averse to reflecting on, or analysing, what she does, but rather that she believes that practice and theory are mutually sustaining. As Head Nurse at Helen House, her approach has been to lead from alongside not from above; above can, after all, so often mean (or come to mean, as time passes) not a position of superior wisdom and practical experience but one of removal and remoteness.

The gynaecological ward at the Churchill Hospital where Edith worked for eleven years as a staff nurse on night duty was a very busy ward, coping with emergency admissions as well as with patients admitted for surgery. It was on this ward that Edith met Sister Benedicta who had been admitted for treatment of ovarian cancer. Two long conversations Edith had with Benedicta changed the pattern of her (and her family's) life dramatically. It was Benedicta's noticing the Alder Hey Children's Hospital badge that Edith was wearing that first led her to talk to Edith about children's nursing and then to mention Helen House. When Benedicta suggested that Edith should apply for the job of Head Nurse at Helen House, Edith brushed the suggestion aside, saying that half the nurses in Oxford would be applying for the job and in any case she was too old to be considered. Benedicta's response was simple – 'Rubbish!' She told Edith to write to Mother Frances and ask to meet her. This Edith did, in March 1982.

At that first meeting between Edith and Frances, Frances described what she saw as the role of Helen House and explained how she envisaged the hospice working. Edith, for her part, said that she was now at a stage when she could envisage working full time and that she would be prepared to work at Helen House for between five and seven years, that is to say until her husband retired. What she was interested in and wanted to be involved in, was hands-on nursing which is why she was not interested in the Head Nurse post which Frances had by now suggested she should seriously consider; at that stage, perhaps because of her experience to date, she presumably saw the role of Head Nurse as more an administrative, than an active nursing, one.

Frances said that she would be in touch after the Head Nurse had been appointed. Edith saw the advertisement for the post of Head Nurse duly appear in the *Nursing Times* and waited to hear about subsequent interviews with the newly-appointed Head Nurse for nursing staff. However, when Frances again rang her as promised, it was to say that she was sending her an application form for the post of Head Nurse. Edith completed the form and was asked to come to an interview with Frances, Heather de Freitas and Roger Burne. By this time she felt she would love to have the job of Head Nurse but she still felt unable to believe it would ever be hers. Perhaps this feeling led her to be very straightforward and certainly uncalculating and slightly unguarded in her answers to questions put to her at her interview. She describes how she did not give any of the 'right' answers but simply said what she believed and felt. It is cheering to think that Edith was chosen as Head Nurse on the basis of what she honestly felt and believed, that the three people who interviewed her recognized that Edith's beliefs and feelings *were* 'the right answers'.

Edith took up her post of Head Nurse two months before Helen House opened. This was extremely helpful because it meant that she and Pip Leitch, who was appointed Deputy Head Nurse in the early autumn, were around to provide the 'nurse's perspective' on the final details in the equipping of Helen House. Their input even (or especially) at this late stage, was invaluable.

Another advantage of Edith being around in the months before Helen House opened was that she was able, with Frances, to interview and appoint staff in an unhurried, thorough and thoughtful manner. She was able to meet people on more than one occasion if that seemed sensible and she was able to talk to them at length and begin to get to know them. She was also able to identify people whom she felt would be able to work together well and to achieve a good balance of professional and human skills in her staff team. It was not necessary to advertise for staff to work at Helen House; from the moment the Helen House project was first mentioned publicly and featured in the press and on the radio, Frances had received letters and telephone calls from people interested in working there and after the ITV documentary the steady stream of letters had become a veritable cascade! Frances had filed all the letters and enquiries and it was from these that the original team of fifteen staff was selected.

A House Called Helen

Contrary to what is believed by some, Helen House is staffed neither by nuns nor exclusively by trained nurses, nor is there a doctor permanently in the hospice. You would not necessarily even clap eyes on Frances if you came to stay for a few days, for her many other commitments and duties mean that long periods of time can sometimes elapse without her being able to be at Helen House. Incidentally, contrary to what some of the more sentimental outpourings in the popular papers would have you believe, papers which, far from being economical with the truth are amazingly generous in the way they expand it and embroider on it, you might have to wait a long time before your visit coincided with a visit by H.R.H. The Duchess of Kent!

Helen House is staffed by a team of salaried staff who bring to their job a variety of skills and talents. In the current Helen House brochure, the paragraph headed 'Who works in Helen House?' begins with the sentence: 'Helen House is run by people whose common qualification is their love and concern for children'. The staff at Helen House are such a varied group of individuals, each with his or her particular gifts, skills and personality, that to provide any meaningful and apt collective description of them is difficult without, if you are not careful, resorting to describing what they are *not*, rather than what they *are*. When the original brochure was updated, about five years after Helen House opened, Richard and I put forward the sentence quoted above as a positive description of the team which puts the emphasis on what they offer rather than on what they do not try to offer. Frances has described the ideal staff member of Helen House as being 'a card-carrying member of the human race'. Professional skills are no substitute for humanity and empathy in the context of Helen House. This is not to say that professional skills are discounted or undervalued, but rather that when staff are appointed their 'human' qualities, quite as much as their professional expertise, are borne in mind. As it happens, in addition to the trained nurses you would expect to find among the staff members, there are other individuals with professional qualifications; the present Deputy Head is a trained teacher and the team includes a physiotherapist, a social worker and a nursery nurse. What it is important to remember, though, is that their professional skills (even in the case of the nurses) were not the only reason they were offered their jobs at Helen House. A high level of professional nursing expertise is needed though not all the time by all the children as, by contrast, concern, interest, empathy and human warmth *are* – and these are needed by the families too. It cannot be stressed too often that the starting point for Helen House was a human one not a medical one and that it is humanity that sustains the hospice.

The staff at Helen House do not wear uniform. They are, after all, temporarily replacing, or acting on behalf of, the parents, friends, brothers and sisters and relatives of the ill child who care for him or her at home. Helen House is concerned with people helping people. One member of the team says that what he particularly enjoys about working there is the feeling that he is part of a caring team which includes the family and the child. As he puts it, there is no 'them and us' feeling. Because they do not have uniforms, staff are aware that they cannot, to quote Edith, 'hide behind their badge or qualifications'. They cannot rest on their laurels, looking back to qualifications earned in the past to affirm their present status or skill. Their position, their ability to help, is affirmed (or weakened) afresh with each day that passes; they stand (or fall) continually, depending on how they approach and support a child and his family. They can no more rest on past successes than can footballers; to quote the manager of Oxford United, 'It's every day, every match.'

As regards the day-to-day running of Helen House, role-sharing is the approach that has obtained since the hospice opened and which enhances the home-from-home atmosphere. Basically, everybody does everything (with the exception of measuring of drug doses and a few medical procedures which can only be undertaken by a doctor or qualified nurse). Team members working on a shift might find themselves cooking, cleaning, playing with children, taking children for walks or on excursions, tidying the kitchen cupboards, cleaning the windows, having a jacuzzi with a child, talking to families; they have to be prepared to do whatever is needed or seems most important at that particular time. Incidentally, this applies quite as much to the Head Nurse as to any other team member; Edith is by no means desk-bound and while I have often seen her pushing a hoover around I have never seen her armed with a clipboard. The fact that role-sharing applies across the board, not just at some levels, indeed the fact that the word 'level' seems inappropriate in this context, is something that is greatly appreciated by the team. The staff organization at Helen House is democratic, not hierarchical.

Most people are probably familiar with jokes about hospital life of the sort, 'Wake up, Mr Jones, it's time for your sleeping tablets'. In a large institution such as a hospital, where you are coping with very large numbers of patients and often operating with limited staff, it is probably necessary, in order to ensure the smooth running of the establishment, to have oft-affirmed rules and a fairly rigid timetable. Sometimes, sadly, but perhaps inevitably, inflexibility sets in and an individual patient's comfort can be put, unnecessarily, second to the smooth running of the machine. Because Richard and I remembered a few painful instances of this from when Helen was in hospital for six months and because, in any case, Helen House was not intended in any way to mirror a hospital or institution, we had always said from the outset that there would be no rules at Helen House; the only rule was that there should be no rules. Of course, there are a few basic safety rules, but these would obtain anywhere where people take a responsible attitude to life. There are no rules (as there sometimes are in institutions) whose sole purpose would seem to be to draw a distinguishing line between those in positions of power and having superior knowledge and those over whom they exercise that power and whom they seek to intimidate with that knowledge.

A parent, for example, might know that a warm milky drink at midnight was immensely soothing to their child and might ask the staff at Helen House to provide that. The Helen House staff would accept that the parent obviously knows the child best and would try to provide the drink the child particularly liked. There would be no danger of the parent being told that the drinks trolley went round at 8.30 pm and after that the rule was no hot drinks until 6.00 am! Such flexibility is obviously much easier in a small and intimate setting than in a large institution but it is not a by-product exclusively of small scale; attitudes enter into it to a great extent, too.

Such 'rules' as there are, are not ones of which children and parents would necessarily even be aware. There has to be at least one qualified nurse on each shift and he or she holds the keys to the drugs cupboard and is responsible for measuring drug doses. Other 'rules' are dictated by common sense rather than by a need to bolster a hierarchical structure. One such rule is that volunteers do not answer the phone. This is clearly sensible, since many of the volunteers are not in Helen House often enough to get to know the set-up intimately and thus to be able to answer the questions a caller might put to them. Another 'rule' is that if a team member is going out with a child for a walk or shopping they must tell the person in charge of the shift; the whereabouts of all staff on duty must be known at all times. Other 'rules' have their foundation in safety considerations tempered by humanity; an example is the 'rule' that no sick child is ever left on his or her own or at least where a team member cannot keep an eye on him or her and offer assistance or comfort if necessary.

Certain things are simply understood and do not need to be enshrined in regulatory language. One such thing is that meal times are social occasions and the staff eat with the children. Another, much more fundamental, guiding principle is that answers to children's questions should be simple, direct and truthful. This is obviously something which is discussed with parents but the aim is never to lie, pretend or deceive.

Perhaps if we say that the only rule peculiar to Helen House is that the well-being, in its widest sense, of ill children and their families and of everyone involved in their care is paramount, we have said it all.

In addition to the day-to-day jobs which are shared by all the team members equally, there are specific, less frequently recurring but on-going, jobs which have to be done. A few examples are shopping for food and cleaning materials etc.; interviewing prospective volunteers and keeping the rota of volunteers up-to-date and running smoothly; and tidying, cataloguing and maintaining the many tapes and videos that Helen House has for visiting children's use. These specific tasks are allocated to individual members of the team who perhaps particularly enjoy them or are particularly good at them. All such allocation of duties and responsibilities is negotiable and can be reviewed whenever wished.

The Helen House day is organized around three shifts – 7.30 am to 3.00 pm, 1.30 pm to 9.30 pm and 9.00 pm to 8.00 am. 'Hand-over' occurs at 7.30 am, 1.30 pm and 9.00 pm, and during hand-over the person in charge of the outgoing shift makes sure that those coming on duty know anything they might need to know about the children in their care. In addition to information passed on in conversation – how well individual children are eating and sleeping, whether they have had any fits or similar problems, whether they are in good spirits, what, if any, activities they have enjoyed – team members going off duty record in the individual notes of the child they have been looking after anything relating to his or her care that those who will be caring for him or her on the next or subsequent shifts might find it helpful to know.

The person in charge of a shift, the person who holds the keys, is always a qualified nurse. Where it happens that there are two qualified nurses on the same shift, which of them is in charge is decided entirely democratically; the one who is in charge is the one who was most recently on a shift. If this still does not throw up a 'winner' then it is left to the nurses to decide the matter between themselves.

There are usually six or seven team members on each daytime shift. At night there are two members of staff on duty but these two can 'draft in' extra staff as required. As befits the democratic set-up at Helen House, they are left with considerable discretion in this; if they feel, for whatever reason, that they need additional staff, they can ring up and bring them in. This can be done some time in advance – for example, if the night staff notice that a child, or several children, requiring extra supervision or whose condition means that they make particular demands on the staff, are booked to come and stay – or on the spur of the moment, as a difficult, or potentially difficult, situation arises. The basic core of night staff work only at night; they are not the same staff who are in Helen House during the day, but they are long-standing members of staff, and parents and children get to know them well. When they draft in extra help they do so from a 'bank' of people known to Helen House, or they ask one of the day-time team to help out. Several of the day-time staff are very happy to do the occasional night shift where this does not undermine their ability to carry out their day-time duties. Incidentally, the night staff regularly wash the kitchen, bathroom and lavatory floors and tidy the linen cupboard when necessary, during the night shift – jobs that are not always practicable during a busy day with (often) active children around.

When staff were appointed initially, Edith was able to be very flexible and to meet the specific requirements of individual team members relating to working hours and time off. For example, to begin with she felt able to employ staff who, for family reasons, wished to work from 9.00 am to 2.00 pm every day but not to work shifts. Although flexibility still exists where possible, the growing number of children and families coming to Helen House has meant that it has, inevitably, had to be reduced somewhat and all the Helen House team now work the standard shift pattern.

A House Called Helen

Most of the people who work on the team at Helen House are women. It is interesting to reflect on why this is so. Perhaps, as is often said, women are, by nature, drawn to this sort of 'nurturing' work. Perhaps it has something to do with the attitudes of society; what are considered the caring and nurturing roles in society are seen to be the province of women. Undoubtedly, the initial flexibility in working hours at Helen House suited women wanting to combine part-time (but challenging) work with bringing up children and being at home when their children were at home, so this is one obvious reason for the 'gender imbalance' in the Helen House team. Perhaps the most telling fact is that there is no career structure in place at Helen House and there are no obvious promotion prospects, which means that to work there you need to be unambitious in terms of professional advancement though hugely ambitious in terms of 'human effectiveness'. Also, you have to accept that you will never be a high earner. We live in a society where in general, despite some changes in attitude, men are still esteemed (or at least slotted in to the 'successful' or 'unsuccessful' category) largely on the basis of their earning power. The difference in attitudes to men and women is clear from even a cursory reading of newspapers. A woman in the news is described in terms of her person and her role in relation to other people ('Vivacious, forty-four-year-old mother-of-three'); a man is described in terms of his financial status ('Speaking from his £250,000 Victorian house in a sought-after suburb of the city . . .'). In such a climate it must be difficult for men who might perhaps wish to do so to take on a job that is not financially well-rewarded (because, traditionally, it has been seen as a woman's job!).

The staff at Helen House refer to themselves as 'the team': 'I work on the team'; 'Have you met the new member of the team?'; 'The team feels that the carpet in the playroom needs replacing'. I have to confess that to begin with Richard and I found the word 'team' rather off-putting, perhaps because, with its sporting associations, it had rather hearty connotations

142

for us. Also the word 'team' is so often used nowadays in all sorts of business organizations and places of work to suggest a purposeful, united and therefore effective approach, where nothing has been done in real terms to bring the people in the so-called 'team' together and make them feel they have a common aim and all have something to contribute. Thus it is often, in a sense, a cover-up, a mere paying of lip-service to laudable ideals. Happily, we have come to accept (and use willingly) the word team to describe the staff at Helen House because of the way the staff work; they do have a common goal and, like the members of a good sports team, they clearly all contribute equally to the team's success. Very importantly, they are all seen to be, and are treated as being, of equal worth.

In the context of Helen House the word 'team' to describe the staff is actually very apt. The use of the word draws attention to the importance of co-operation. The team members have to espouse the aims of Helen House. This does not mean that they shed their individuality, but rather that they channel that individuality into serving the common aim. Significantly, new staff members, however promising they may appear as individuals at interview, are never appointed before they have worked a shift at Helen House alongside other team members. Their appointment then remains provisional until they have served a probationary period (usually of six months) and shown that they can in fact operate as part of a team. They then receive a contract.

The team spirit at Helen House is reinforced not only by shared social activities (for example an annual party coinciding roughly with Helen House's birthday in November and an annual excursion or 'away day') but on a more regular and formal basis by meetings. There is usually a one-hour staff meeting once a week, presided over by the Head Nurse or Deputy Head although this is cancelled if the hospice is particularly busy or the demands of the visiting children make a break for discussion seem inappropriate. At this meeting anything relating to the smooth day-to-day running of Helen

House, at whatever level, can be discussed. Anybody can put anything on the agenda, provided it is something relevant to how Helen House operates or should operate. Edith might choose to remind the team of the importance of punctuality; a team member might wish to introduce the topic of cleaning and remind the others that they are all supposed to share this exciting task! Sometimes seemingly minor details can lead to an animated discussion about the philosophy of Helen House. What is important is that the weekly staff meeting is a democratic forum for discussion aimed at strengthening the effectiveness of the Helen House team (and thereby of what Helen House was set up to do). A recent innovation at the weekly staff meetings is the short talk given on occasion by a team member. Team members have taken it in turns to find out as much as they can about a particular (often rare) illness, usually one that a child they care for at Helen House is suffering from and in which they, therefore, have a particular interest, and have then 'presented' this information to the rest of the team.

In addition to the staff meeting at which more obviously practical and administrative matters are discussed there is another weekly staff meeting at which less tangible subjects come up. From the outset, when Helen House was first mooted, there was recognition of the fact that the work that staff would be doing, while it would probably be challenging, fulfilling and possibly even exciting, would be harrowing. The potential stress on staff of working with, and growing to love, children whose life span was limited, of witnessing and sharing the pain this caused those children's families – this stress was recognized very early on and it was felt that there should be some regular forum in which the team could discuss their feelings and give and receive support. This forum is provided by a weekly meeting in the middle of the day, attended by all the team members on duty that day, on whatever shift. (Cover for staff attending this meeting is provided by other members of the team who are drafted in on a regular basis.) At this meeting staff discuss their feelings about any aspect whatsoever of their work, whether in Helen House or outside as they develop friendships with families in a wider context. They talk about difficulties they may have and of how they work with, and identify with, each other. Some of the team find such 'soul-baring' difficult and choose not to say much; others find great relief in having an opportunity to air problems they are having and get other people's views on these. The meeting is not intended as a forum for staff to discuss personal problems completely unrelated to their role at Helen House, but apart from this proviso it offers the chance for no-holds-barred discussion. Some of the team members say that even if they do not feel they wish to speak up much, they have found it very illuminating and helpful to learn of the (perhaps completely unsuspected) views and feelings of their colleagues. To begin with, the meeting was led by Dr Gillian Forrest, a child psychiatrist from the Park Hospital, whom by chance Richard and I had met on our visit to Bradwell Grove and who has given generously and regularly of her time to support this worthwhile venture. Latterly the meeting has at times been organized by Helen Woolley, a family and child guidance worker, who also offers personal one-to-one support sessions for staff on one day a week at which staff are free to raise any matters whatsoever, whether related to their work at Helen House or not.

Guidelines laid down by the UK Central Council for Nursing, Midwifery and Health Visiting, relating to training of nurses, say that nurses should undertake five days' training in every three-year period. This is part of PREP – the post-registration education project. The staff at Helen House (whether trained nurses or not) have always been encouraged to go on courses which will help them in their work, either by updating their basic nursing skills or by broadening their knowledge of the nature, progress, pattern and treatment of the illnesses the children they care for at Helen House may be suffering from. In addition to this and to occasional talks from visiting professionals, one week a year is set aside for reflection and for talks and workshops on whatever aspects of their work at Helen House the staff feel it would be helpful to look at more closely or learn more about. This week is usually in November, round about Helen House's birthday. Helen House is closed for respite care (although it remains open for emergencies) and is given a thorough spring (autumn!) cleaning and, when necessary, the decoration is touched up or renewed and maintenance jobs carried out. While this cleaning is going on and the fabric of the building is being spruced up, staff have a chance to stand back from their work and give their ideas a thorough dusting-down and going-over. They speak very positively of this week as giving them a chance not only to think about the broader issues related to their day-to-day caring work and to get a broader perspective, but to recharge their batteries and refresh their attitudes through reflection and unhurried discussion. They also have time to consider anew the aims of Helen House. As one member of staff puts it, 'We all need reminding regularly what the philosophy is.' There is usually a social event on one evening of this week. In the year of Helen House's fifth birthday we invited all the staff and their partners to a party in our home. It was a very happy occasion when all the staff of Helen House came to Helen's house.

Talking to the staff at Helen House about how they see their job, what they enjoy about working at Helen House and what causes stress throws up a number of oft-recurring themes. Though the words they use to describe their work inevitably vary, the basic aspirations and ideas are remarkably consistent. Staff speak of coming alongside children and families as a friend; they speak of reducing fear (in both children and their relatives) and reducing the sense of isolation that engulfs so many families with a very sick child; more generally they speak of caring and more obviously of removing pain. In a variety of different ways, members of the team speak of sharing the load that Helen House families bear, both the physical and the emotional load.

In sharing the emotional load you obviously make yourself vulnerable to the emotions in question. Sharing is such an overworked and abused word nowadays, often meaning little more than telling somebody something, relaying some basic fact to another person, that the empathy and giving of oneself that is involved in any true sharing (anything above the level of dividing up a chocolate bar, let us say!) are increasingly devalued or forgotten. The staff at Helen House recognize that in sharing the emotional pain of the families who come to Helen House they cannot themselves remain impervious to that pain; indeed, they recognize that feeling that pain themselves in some measure is inevitable and necessary if they are to offer any real help or comfort. 'The day you're not affected, you get out', as one team member puts it.

Describing what they like about their job at Helen House, team members say they enjoy working with people and enjoy the company and friendship both of the children and families who come to Helen House and of the other members of the team. They greatly enjoy the support they get from their colleagues on the team; though they feel they give a lot, they also feel they receive a lot and that the support team members give each other extends beyond the working environment. One team member, in fact, speaks of the 'supportive and therapeutic atmosphere' at Helen House as being 'a fringe benefit of working here'.

One member of the team speaks enthusiastically of the 'unhurried nature of the day' at Helen House and of how you feel you have time for the things that matter – cuddling the children, talking to families, sharing a joke. She attributes this to the size of Helen House and feels that if the hospice were bigger, staff might feel less relaxed and more bound by the constraints of time than directed by the needs of individuals. If there were simply more people around, the atmosphere would change. As an example of this, she points to the change in atmosphere at Helen House during the 'change-over' period when you have, temporarily, members of two shifts in the

147

building. She describes the atmosphere then as 'too bustly' and says that the increased numbers lead to tension.

As you would expect, members of the Helen House team attribute much of their job satisfaction to the feeling that they are doing something worthwhile. They derive satisfaction from helping people whose needs are all too often overlooked. Moreover, they feel cheered and strengthened by the affirmation of human values which is what Helen House is all about. This affirmation comes in the adherence at Helen House to the belief that, though staff cannot cure the terrible illness of a child, they still have much to offer that child and his family; they can ease the family's pain by simply being with them in their suffering, by feeling both for, and with, them. The restorative power of human warmth, love and compassion is immense and receiving them is often what gives families the strength to go on, whether before or after their child has died.

Interestingly, when they talk about what they find stressful about their work, the team do not usually point to the closeness of death, or to their feelings on the death of a child, as a common trigger of stress. More mundane things such as interpersonal relations within the team are more often pinpointed. Interestingly, such stress as minor disagreements or malaise with colleagues may cause, evaporates when a child dies at Helen House. As one team member puts it, 'We all come together then and feel very close; nothing is too much trouble.' However, though dealing with death itself is not seen as a cause of stress, the problems of serious illness *are*. For example, staff speak of how the tension rises and how they feel under stress if for any reason they are not able to control a child's symptoms, to control his or her pain. Seeing a child suffering is something they find very distressing. Another thing staff find very difficult is watching a child deteriorate, often over a period of months and years. To see a child who perhaps initially, though afflicted by a serious illness, could walk and talk, laugh and play, gradually slip into a state of total helplessness is very painful. The hardest part of the job is watching families come back time after time and seeing the deterioration in their child. 'I find it so hard watching families lose another little bit of the child', one team member told me.

I think that job satisfaction at Helen House is greatly enhanced by the democratic set-up, by the total absence of a rigid hierarchical structure jacked up by rules for the sake of rules. This democratic set-up fosters a feeling of self-worth among the staff. Each individual team member can feel that his or her view is as valid as the next person's. Many of the best decisions are, after all, based on instinct, many of the best actions undertaken on the promptings of the heart. Action based on gut feelings need not be suspect simply because gut feelings cannot be measured or quantified. 'I feel in my bones that it's right' can be the basis for effective and appropriate action, for all its seeming vagueness.

The fact that promotion prospects at Helen House are non-existent because of the lack of a career structure could seem to some to be a problem. However, lack of a career structure has never caused problems with recruitment of staff and has, moreover, had a very positive spin-off. The democratic set-up, where having professional qualifications does not automatically give you any additional clout, does seem to bring out the best in people; it helps people to realize that some things which are perhaps not properly valued in a society where more and more you are esteemed according to your rank, your title and your professional status are in fact of immense worth. The lack of a promotion ladder also encourages individuals to do what they believe in, not what is expedient promotion-wise. This reliance on self and on one's own judgement further increases the individual sense of personal worth, which can only lead to greater effectiveness.

There is no doubt, though, that because the organization of Helen House requires great self-reliance it demands a commensurate confidence in your own instincts, which can take time to develop. The very nature of the complex role the staff assume imposes burdens, too. Unpredictability is the order of the day; staff never know when their skills will be called upon most insistently, nor indeed which skills. They have to hold themselves in readiness, for exactly *what* is never certain. This requires a good measure of adaptability. Since their role will be defined by each individual family and its needs (and these will be as different as individuals are different) what they have to do, essentially, is keep themselves, and all that they are, always available. This requires much greater self-acceptance than is required in a job whose main duties can be starkly and precisely listed.

One team member told me that when she first started working at Helen House, although all the team have got the same role, she felt at a disadvantage because she was not a trained nurse. She felt she often knew what would help a child (physically or 'spiritually') but hesitated, without the backup of professional expertise to support her instinct, to advance her feelings. As she put it, 'It's harder to stand your ground on instinct'. However, she says that the emphasis placed at Helen House on the well-being of each individual child and on the parents as the experts (because of their emotional bond) in caring for that child, has emboldened her in this respect, and she now feels more secure to follow her instincts.

The present climate in our society, however, makes this harder than it might be in different circumstances. We live in a society where you are judged by what you do, not by what you are, where your professional label is more important than where you are as a human being. 'What do you do?' is often one of the opening questions we put to a person we are meeting for the first time at a social gathering; we do not feel at ease with, nor, indeed, start to relate to, a person whom we have not managed to 'place' job-wise. Allied to this is the way that we undervalue common sense, instinct and humanity – or rather we only value them fully if they have been repackaged (often in convoluted language) to sound professional or simply posh. It is little wonder that in this climate those with no professional qualifications (however flimsy or precariously-based the qualifications of the people they compare themselves with may be) often lack confidence in themselves and can feel useless, even if they have great qualities. The worth of what they do instinctively is not recognized (no more by themselves than by others) because it springs from 'mere' common sense.

If you want a simple idea to gain credence and authority, dress it up to sound grand (and, preferably, abstract). Richard and I have come to describe this as the 'formalizing of common sense'. It is amazingly widespread, particularly, sadly, in the fields of education and health care. More and more, people shun the simple and straightforward, favouring instead high-flown abstract language or simply lots of approximate words where one robust one would do. This, they believe, gives an idea more authority.

It would seem that this is not new; more than a century ago Charles Dickens touched on the way that, in a desire to impress, people allow the words they use to convey an idea, to swamp that idea. 'People', he wrote, 'enjoy themselves mightily' when there are 'several good words in succession for the expression of one idea.' Elaborating on this, Dickens continued: 'We talk about the tyranny of words, but we like to tyrannize over them too; we are fond of having a large superfluous establishment of words to wait upon us on great occasions; we think it looks important, and sounds well. As we are not particular about the meaning of our liveries on state occasions, if they be but fine and numerous enough, so, the meaning or necessity of our words is a secondary consideration, if there be but a great parade of them.' He warned that we have 'got into many great difficulties and will get into many greater from maintaining too large a retinue of words'.

Perhaps the worst thing about the growing fashion for using abstract language even when talking about starkly material things, and for avoiding saying things in a direct way, is that it can have the effect in the long run of eroding the impact of the simple idea within the (abstract) packaging, of making it lose its immediacy and, indeed, its meaning. Real communication soon becomes very difficult. Perhaps I could give an illustration of this.

Helen is totally helpless. The effects of the operation she had on her brain many years ago were devastating. We have to do everything for her. We love her dearly and we look after her at home. We organize our lives so as to care for Helen as well as we possibly can and at the same time to cater for the needs of her sisters and to live as full, interesting and rich a life as we can ourselves. This is not easy but we never expected it to be. We never feel we do enough for Helen and we will never give up thinking about how we might manage things better. To say that Helen, in all her helplessness and with all her problems, is looked after at home I believe immediately gets across some idea of her, and our, difficulties. To say that (I quote) 'she is in receipt of a care package in the home situation' (quite apart from suggesting a degree of outside help which has not been our experience) does not.

People often ask us about Helen House and how it operates. One of the things we find hardest to get across to people is that very ill children come to stay at Helen House for short periods while their families or those looking after them have a break. That the success of Helen House stems in large part from its providing practical help in a straightforward manner is something many people simply cannot grasp. The idea behind Helen House seems too simple to be credible! Perhaps we have become so accustomed to being served ideas and facts heavily larded with jargon and complicated abstract theory that we find it hard to digest simple fare?

Because Helen House is concerned with helping children with life-threatening illness and because it is called a hospice (which for many people has connotations of imminent death) people often imagine that death must be ever in the air at Helen House, that the atmosphere must be immensely depressing. But though (or perhaps because) the staff know that the children who come to stay at Helen House cannot look forward to a long life, they place the emphasis very firmly on enhancing the quality of whatever life these children may still have ahead of them. Affirmation of life even in the face of death is one of the things Helen House is most involved in.

When interviewing potential new members of staff, Edith is at pains to make this clear and always stresses to possible new team members that Helen House is not eight children lying in bed dying! In this context it is helpful to remember that a child with a life-threatening illness may be ill over many years and not necessarily even obviously so for all of those years. The word 'hospice' leads many people to believe that all the children who come to Helen House are in the last stages of a terminal illness, whereas in fact many of the children come for respite care, at regular or irregular intervals, throughout what is often a protracted and only slowly incapacitating illness. Throughout this illness, however long or short it may turn out to be, the staff at Helen House aim not only to ease any pain or discomfort the children may experience and to reduce fear, but also to increase opportunities for enjoyment and happiness, to help the children live life to the full, in terms of intensity if not of length.

The atmosphere within Helen House is certainly not one of unremitting gloom. The atmosphere and character changes from one day to the next and, in fact, is determined very greatly by which children and families are staying at any particular time. Sometimes the mood is more reflective and Helen House very quiet; sometimes, if an ill child who also happens to be quite noisy and active is staying (or even several of them) the noise level rises dramatically. The sort of activities, entertainment and conversation different children and, indeed, different families enjoy inevitably affects the atmosphere; some people (whether ill or not) are simply more vocally sociable than others!

One thing that never changes, or rather is constantly under review, is the quality of the environment. Helen House is very much lived in and inevitably this means there has been a certain amount of wear and tear on the building and equipment. Every effort is made to keep the decoration in good condition and to replace things that have begun to look tatty. Just as we felt at the outset that the quality of the environment was very important for staff and visiting children and families alike, so now, years on, we feel that no effort should be spared in maintaining that quality. As one member of the team puts it, though some people might think the provision could be more basic, the high-quality environment gives a message to the sick children and their families who turn to Helen House – you are valued. This is a message that many of them receive all too seldom.

Perhaps because they, too, feel valued, staff have tended to stay. Over the years since Helen House opened there has been a very low staff turnover; at the end of the first ten years the key posts were still occupied by their original incumbents, with the exception of the post of Deputy Head. (When Pip Leitch left the area she was replaced in 1987 by Eve Herd whose appointment meant an interesting change of role for her; she had previously worked as secretary in the Helen House office.) Where staff have left this has usually been because their family was moving away or because they were getting married and leaving the area or because they were, in any case, for a specific reason, on a short-term contract; perhaps they had come to Helen House for a year as part of their training before embarking on a Health Visitor's course or because they were wives of ordinands training in Oxford. Generally, staff have not wanted to leave, nor has it seemed appropriate that they should. It is sometimes said that two years working in a hospice is the maximum possible; the job is thought to be too emotionally draining for anyone to do it for longer. That the staff at Helen House have not found this to be the case is interesting. The strength of the mutual support between team members is significant, as is the fact that Helen House is small and that there is a balance between respite care (albeit of very ill children) and terminal care. Whereas in a hospice which concentrates on terminal care you might regularly have several deaths a week, this is rare at Helen House. The fact that usually time elapses between deaths means that the team have time, as one of them puts it, to 'renew themselves' and to talk and share feelings.

Before Helen House actually opened, everybody connected with it had been involved in the public side, fund-raising, giving talks, talking to interested parties. When it opened the 'private' side had to establish an identity of its own, which took time, and at the same time the office, under Mike Garside, became the 'public front' of Helen House. Mike not only undertook from the start all the administrative work at Helen House (dealing with staff salaries, bills, supplies of equipment etc.) but his was the voice that would usually speak first to any caller on the telephone and the face that any visitor to Helen House would usually first see. The Helen House office is at the front of the building, with windows looking out both on to the garden at the side and on to the paved area at the front and the entrance gate. Visitors calling, perhaps to bring donations of money or toys or fruit or whatever, or to buy notelets or to pick up covenant forms, would almost invariably meet Mike. He also took calls from newspapers and fielded questions from people curious to know more. In a sense, Mike has always taken the flak – for example when people have been unable to grasp the simple truth that Helen House is, for obvious reasons, a private place, a place where families and children can enjoy peace and privacy and not a place that casual visitors can look round; when callers have felt that their undoubtedly kind and much appreciated donation entitled them to a guided tour; or when he has rightly turned away press or television photographers wanting intimate pictures inside Helen House to support a feature. When visitors come to Helen House, their business may not require them to go further than the main office. If a long conversation is necessary, this takes place in the discussion room, the only other room (apart from a small cloakroom) opening off the main entrance hall. The 'private' side of Helen House begins beyond a door at the back of the entrance hall and this door is not open to casual or 'business' visitors.

At the same time as the two parts of Helen House – the private and the public – were establishing their separate identities, Frances's role was changing. As the team at Helen House increasingly took on the private, 'human' role, coming alongside families with very ill children and offering friendship, support and help, Frances's role became an increasingly public one. Moreover, her public was no longer usually the general public; increasingly she was meeting and talking to groups of professionals. She was much in demand as a speaker at medical conferences and seminars and on religious retreats and ministry training courses. Increasingly often she addressed audiences of doctors, nurses, social workers and health care professionals. Although the starting point for Helen House had been a human, not a medical, one, and it had been human experience and feeling, not professional judgement, that had pointed to the need for it and determined its form, the service Helen House offered was one which the medical profession, and the caring professions generally, realized they needed to know about, cutting as it did across the boundaries between the areas of care they in their different professions were involved in. Frances recognized the great importance of explaining the work of Helen House to as wide an audience as possible; since Helen House was the first children's hospice in the country and might therefore be seen as the obvious 'model' for any future provision, it was important that the philosophy behind it and the way it operated should be clearly understood. Another important reason for Frances giving so much of her time to talking to professionals was the need to dispel suspicion and mistrust and to strengthen professional confidence. Doctors and other professionals are used to being in a position of control over their patients or clients and do not always take readily to sending them for help or support outside the boundaries of their profession or allied professions.

After the Opening

The months after Helen House opened were a very lonely time for Richard and me. For more than two years we had been working towards the opening of Helen House and had devoted much of our creative energy to its planning. Inevitably there was a sense almost of anticlimax when suddenly our hopes were realized, even if, of course, a new goal – that of ensuring that Helen House operated as intended and remained true to its ideals – immediately emerged. We saw very little of Frances, for the reasons given above, and initially we saw little of the team at Helen House. This was because we felt (perhaps wrongly) that we should leave them alone for a while, to settle in to their role and because, too, we were aware of the ambiguity in our position *vis-à-vis* the staff which might make them, at least to start with, feel rather awkward. Helen was *the* Helen who had inspired the place they now worked in and whose needs had provided the model for the type of care Helen House would provide. Richard and I, while parents of a sick child and therefore potentially typical targets for their concern and help, were also very close friends of Frances and also, as fellow planners with her, very much on the 'administration and staff' side of Helen House. We did not wish the staff to think we expected special treatment for Helen because she was who she was and we were who we were. We did not want the staff to think we were watching them to see if they were doing their job properly. We held back and did not approach Helen House. The staff, perhaps thinking that we did not need their services probably because (how often this has created problems for us!) we seemed to cope so well, did not make a move towards us. Being both potential receiver and provider gave us problems in those early days; we were immensely lonely, because we could operate as neither.

Now that the initial awkwardness has entirely dissipated, now that Helen House is so established and the enormous appreciation of those who use it has made the staff much more confident in themselves and their role, the benefit of Richard and me having, so to speak, a foot in both camps, is widely

157

recognized. We are on the receiving end of much of what we were involved in planning and setting up. We know many of the whys and wherefores of the provision, we know what informed the decisions relating to that provision and have discussed these often and, on occasion, at length with Frances, the Head Nurse, the Medical Director and the Administrator; equally, we, along with the other parents who bring their children to Helen House, seek support and help from the team and comfort in the atmosphere. We, like the other parents, entrust our beloved child to the care of the team at Helen House and we know what it is about the atmosphere that makes us (and them) feel able to do so. We have got to know other parents well and have talked to them about our, and their, feelings. Our situation gives us a unique overview of Helen House, a broader perspective possibly than almost anyone else. Having a foot in both camps means that we can feed information and ideas and thoughts two ways.

Of course, one of the reasons we are in this unique position is because of Helen's continuing life. Despite her increasing frailty, Helen's grip on life is tenacious. When we were planning Helen House, I do not think either Richard or I envisaged actually using Helen House ourselves; we believed we were providing something that might help other families in situations similar to ours in the future. In what might seem our more fanciful moments, we sometimes felt that Helen might quite simply fade away as soon as Helen House opened; that she was clinging on to life to oversee the founding of 'her house', but that, once her mission was accomplished, she would quietly die.

The reality proved to be very different. Helen House opened and Helen lived on, helpless, frail, but with a strange aura of dignity and serenity. She continued to inspire great love and by us, certainly, she was loved beyond measure. That she should be so frail, when what had sprung from her helplessness was daily growing in strength, was poignant.

Ever since I had first met Frances and had told her about

Helen's illness, a candle had been kept burning, day and night, in the window of the chapel at All Saints Convent, accompanied at all times, even in the depths of winter, by a small bunch of fresh flowers provided, and lovingly arranged, by one of the sisters, Sister Helen Irene. At night the light from the candle was clearly visible across the convent garden, shining out in the darkness. One day, around the time Helen House opened, Frances asked me rather tentatively if I thought the time had come for the candle to be put out. I think I had probably always imagined that the candle would burn so long as Helen was still alive, that it would be put out only when her life was extinguished. A wave of pain swept over me, but passed as suddenly as it had come. I told Frances the time had indeed come. Helen House now stood in place of that candle, as a beacon of light in the darkness, multiplying the power of that candle a million times over. As I said to Frances, 'The light has moved across the garden.'

7

The Philosophy at Work

Though Helen's life provided the spark from which the idea of Helen House was kindled, the idea which then sprang into vigorous and blazing life – her life, in contrast to what usually happens to the match that lights the fire, did not go out as the fire took hold. Helen House opened and was soon to be cited as a shining example of how gravely-ill children and their families could be cared for and supported. It was to blaze a trail in the provision of hospice care for children and young adults. Helen, meanwhile, lived on, her twilight existence the mere embers of the full and cheerful life she had once known and which had been so tragically dampened down.

The first child from a 'Helen House family' to die was a local girl aged ten who suffered from Hurler's Syndrome. She died in Helen House in January 1983. Since Rachel's death, one hundred and seventy-two other children have died out of two hundred and eighty-six who have visited Helen House. (Figures correct up to end of 1992.) Of these children seventy-three (about forty per cent) have died at home, fifty-one (about thirty per cent) at Helen House, thirty-nine (about twenty-five per cent) in hospital and ten (about five per cent) elsewhere (for example at school). Sometimes when a child has died at home, a member of the Helen House team has been with the family in their own home. Almost always when a child has died at Helen House, one of his or her family has been there; often the whole family has been present. On occasion a very ill child has been transferred from hospital to Helen House at the very end of his or her life, at the express wish of the family. The aim is always to do what the family want and find most helpful or easiest to cope with. Care at Helen

House is 'family-driven'.

The illnesses that Helen House children suffer from cover a wide spectrum. Some of the disorders and illnesses are extremely rare; indeed many GPs and nurses might never have heard of them, let alone encountered them among their patients. In a couple of cases, a Helen House child is one of the few known sufferers from an illness in the entire world.

About one in three (thirty per cent) of the two hundred and eighty-six children who have come to Helen House (up to the end of 1992) have suffered from a progressive neurological disease (such as Batten's disease, adrenoleucodystrophy, metachromatic leucodystrophy and Huntington's chorea). About one in five children (twenty-one per cent) have had metabolic defects from birth (such as Hurler's, Sanfilippo or Lowe's syndrome and cystic fibrosis). About one in six children (sixteen per cent) have suffered from neoplasms, of which about a half have been brain tumours and a half other forms of childhood cancer, including leukaemia. Rather fewer (eleven per cent) have suffered from neuromuscular diseases (Duchenne muscular dystrophy, spinal muscular atrophy), while a similar number (thirteen per cent) have suffered from non-progressive neurological disease such as cerebral palsy. Slightly fewer (eight per cent) have suffered from congenital diseases affecting the heart, spina bifida and chromosome disorders. One child has suffered from an auto-immune disease.

However, within these categories the individual symptoms and characteristics of the disease can vary quite widely so that the needs of different children do not fit a set pattern. A large majority of all the children who have come to Helen House have suffered from impaired or total lack of mobility (ninety-five per cent). Three out of four children (seventy-four per cent) have impaired speech or no speech at all, while over one quarter of children (twenty-nine per cent) have impaired vision. Difficulty with feeding is also a common problem (fifty-eight per cent) and digestive problems are frequently encountered. Sometimes very special diets are required. Incontinence (seventy-five per cent) and constipation (forty per cent) are additional problems. Nearly half (forty-two per cent) of the children who have come have suffered from fits or seizures, while over one quarter (thirty-two per cent) have required treatment for pain.

Children come to Helen House from all over the country. While about one sixth of the children who have stayed have come from within a ten mile radius, a similar number have travelled over a hundred miles to get there. About one third of Helen House children have lived between fifty-one and one hundred miles away, with a similar number coming from between eleven and fifty miles away. The families travelling the greatest distance to use Helen House have included three families from Tyne and Wear and four families from Cornwall.

Since it is never easy to travel great distances with a very ill or disabled child, the fact that many families undertake long journeys to reach Helen House is significant. Whether it is an indication of the value they place on what Helen House has to offer, or whether it is an indication of the lack of respite care facilities or support generally, and of the appalling inadequacies of the Community Care system in their home areas, or whether it is a combination of the two, can only be gauged by talking to individual families.

From the outset, flexibility in catering for the needs of the families who turn to Helen House for help was felt to be of paramount importance. For this reason there is no prescribed pattern of respite care, no decreed entitlement to a certain number of days, weekends or whatever. Families decide for themselves what suits them best and best helps them to carry on and continue to bear the burden of long-term caring. When, in the early stages of planning Helen House, we were trying to explain to people what the hospice's role and purpose would be, Richard and I often said that we hoped Helen House would make more families with very ill children feel able to take on the job of caring for their children at home, by providing back-up support, a safety-net always in place (though not necessarily used regularly) to give them confidence as they walked the emotional and practical tightrope that long-term caring so often is. Families in similar situations to our own would not necessarily use Helen House regularly or frequently, but the knowledge that it was there and that they could turn to it for help whenever they felt the need, would be immensely reassuring and might often determine whether they felt able to have their very ill child at home with them (rather than, say, in hospital or institutional care) in the first place. For some families, the simple knowledge that the safety-net was there might be enough in itself to keep them going; for others, the need to test the safety-net regularly and often might be compelling. From this it follows logically that if Helen House is to give support and be of real help to the many very different families who turn to it, it must allow their needs and feelings largely to determine the way they use it. Moreover, the success of Helen House, the importance of what it offers families, cannot be gauged simply by looking at how often these families actually come to the hospice. Statistics could be very misleading here, for Helen House sustains many families in the intangible way that friendship does, and 'what helps us in friendship is not so much the help our friends actually give as the assurance we feel concerning that help.' (Epicurus)

Figures for 1990 show that in that year there were three hundred and forty-eight visits by ill children to Helen House. (Obviously, many of these visits were by the same children returning at various times throughout the year.) Though the length of visits varies, most visits are of less than a week's duration. The average number of times a child or young person comes to stay at Helen House each year is four and the average number of days a child spends at Helen House in a year is twenty-one. Many families might book one quite long visit each year to coincide with their annual holiday, but otherwise visits of more than about two weeks tend to be when the child is very sick rather than for respite. A small number of children come for six or seven days regularly each month.

Probably about one in four families will stay with their child at Helen House. Some will choose to stay at every visit and some choose never to stay, perhaps seeing the time when their child is being looked after at Helen House as a chance to have a complete break, if not from the emotional burden they carry, at least from the practical, and often very physically demanding and draining, burden of day-to-day caring. Some families use Helen House as a base for their holiday or for a rest; they stay in the parents' flat at the front of the building and come and go as they please. Many brothers and sisters of ill children enjoy their holidays at Helen House enormously and clamour to return! Their lively, cheerful presence greatly enhances the family atmosphere that pervades Helen House. The fact that families use the hospice in this way makes Helen House's concern with the affirmation of life, even in the face of crippling, disabling or debilitating illness or of death, very clear. It is not only when their child is most ill that a family will stay at Helen House.

It is immediately clear from looking at the details of children who come to Helen House that not everything has turned out quite as we envisaged in the early planning meetings. In those early days it was thought probable that most of the families using the hospice would come from fairly near Oxford. Because this has not proved to be the case, many of the children coming from some considerable distance, the role of the Medical Director, Roger Burne, has been rather different from what was envisaged. Very few children, probably a maximum of ten over the years, have remained under the care of their own GP while staying at Helen House.

Generally speaking, GPs devolve the care of a child to the Helen House Medical Director. Consequently, Roger is perhaps more closely involved in the day-to-day life of Helen House than he might have envisaged at the outset, an involvement that was enhanced and deepened when, in 1987, he chose to spend part of his six-months' sabbatical leave from his job as a GP at East Oxford Health Centre, working as a member of the team at Helen House. He found this experience invaluable. He says he gained great insight from being closely and actively involved (in a 'hands-on' way) in the day-to-day care of ill children, from getting to know those children as people, as individuals, not simply as medical cases. In a short and very moving report he wrote on his experiences as a member of the care team at Helen House, Roger describes his feelings as he helped to care for one particular child, a twelve-year-old boy with a brain tumour who had been walking and running about twelve months previously and, though increasingly less active, still on his feet and at school only six months before.

Roger was involved in Paul's care for the last two months of the boy's life. During his shifts at Helen House he did for Paul all those things the family of a very ill or helpless child do day in, day out; he washed him, fed him, changed him, cuddled him. At the end of the first afternoon Roger wrote: 'Just an afternoon looking after him and my emotions feel open, raw and vulnerable in a way which is quite different from what happens in my normal work.' When Paul died, Roger felt numb: 'Although I never really knew him, I have washed him, dressed him and looked after him for the last few days.' His feelings of disbelief and then of immense sadness were all the more intense because of his close involvement with Paul over many weeks 'not as a doctor but as a friend.' In the general conclusions he drew from his time on the care team at Helen House, Roger wrote: 'The work is physically exhausting as well as being the most emotional work I have ever done.'

The benefits to everybody, children, families, staff and himself, of the Medical Director having some real understanding of the pressures on the team have proved immense. Roger knows, from personal experience, the demanding and exhausting nature of their work, their recurring feelings of vulnerability and inadequacy and how their growing attachment to, and affection for, the children in their care, makes their work paradoxically both harder and easier.

Because, as time has gone on, Roger has, through his work

165

at Helen House, come into contact with a number of rare disorders and diseases that the average GP might never encounter and, moreover, has seen these conditions in more than one child, he has come to be seen as something of an expert on some of these rare conditions. This is a further reason why he has sometimes become as much involved with the medical care of many of the children who come to Helen House as their own GPs. Aware of the experience Roger has accumulated, parents and GPs themselves have quite naturally turned to him for advice and information on symptom control and treatment generally.

However, the service Roger has offered Helen House from the outset is essentially a GP service. He is not permanently based at the hospice; his main job is as a GP with the nearby Saint Bartholomew's Medical Centre and medical cover for Helen House is a commitment he takes on as a part-time practice commitment (the hospice lies within his practice catchment area). When children come to stay at Helen House, they become temporarily-registered patients of his practice, unless other arrangements are specifically requested (for example for a child to remain under his or her own GP). If anyone at the hospice thinks a particular child should be seen by a doctor, they ring up for a consultation or visit, just as anyone might ring their GP's surgery. However, in order to remain in touch with what is going on at Helen House and to give the team, and indeed children and parents, a chance to get to know him, Roger has always, from the start, organized his working schedule so as to include one regular weekly session at Helen House, a regular time when he is known to be in the hospice and available for discussion, or simply a chat.

Because of the growing numbers of children using Helen House, it became clear (when it had been open for about four years) that Roger needed to be supported in his cover of the hospice by a second doctor. In 1986 Dr Hilary Allinson, a GP from Abingdon who had become closely involved with Helen House through the deaths of two local children who were patients of hers, was appointed to help provide cover and in 1991 another doctor, Ruth Wilson, now a partner at the Temple Cowley Health Centre joined them. (Ruth had been involved with Helen House during her trainee year at Roger's practice.) Between them the three doctors provide medical cover for Helen House. They see this cover as involving more than simply being on call; cover involves being around, 'physically going in to the place'. For this reason, Hilary and Ruth, like Roger, each have a regular weekly session at Helen House. All three doctors are paid for a clinical assistant's session a week to cover this. Each of them does one weekend in three on call. Roger is on call for Helen House during the week, unless he is away from Oxford, in which case Hilary or Ruth are on call, backed up by Roger's practice.

Because the children who come to Helen House have life-threatening illnesses, some people imagine that doctors must be dashing in and out of the hospice all the time, dealing with dramatic problems, and that emergencies must occur with frightening frequency. In fact, this is not the case. The children who come to Helen House are, after all, not children who are receiving acute medical treatment; they are children who are cared for at home by their families, who turn to their GP for help in much the same way as any parent of any child. Of course, medical emergencies do occur from time to time and the doctors can be kept very busy on the occasions when a terminally ill child is staying at Helen House. Getting the symptom control right can be very exacting. However, generally speaking, when a doctor is asked to call, it is, as often as not, for relatively minor things, such as an ear infection, diarrhoea, a touch of asthma. The children staying at Helen House often simply need things any child might need at some time or another.

Strange as it may perhaps seem to some, death is not an emergency at Helen House. As Roger puts it, 'The team can cope with that.' He is not being in any way callous or dismissive or belittling the impact of death on family and friends when he says this; he is according to death its status as an event more human than medical. The parents, relatives and friends of a child who is dying are less likely to request the presence of a doctor (simply because she or he is a doctor) when the child is about to die than they are to request the presence of a member of the Helen House team (and, of course, they may request neither).

Roger, Hilary and Ruth meet regularly at Helen House one lunch time a week to talk about their work and to mull things over. They regard this 'timetabled' coming-together as very important; because they come from three different practices it would be very easy to lose contact with one another. At their meetings they share experiences and sound one another out on issues which might have arisen during the week. There is no fixed agenda though they often discuss individual children and their treatment or, more generally, types of conditions and ways of coping with them. Much of what they do at Helen House is sustained by advance discussion and planning. Their role is not one of sudden crisis management; it is concerned more with ongoing palliative treatment.

As well as overseeing the medical care of children staying at Helen House, the doctors are responsible for admitting a child in the first place, for deciding whether Helen House is appropriate for a child and his or her family and, indeed, whether a child fits into the category of children (and their families) that Helen House was set up to help. Broadly speaking, the criteria for admission which were felt to be right in the planning stage and which were outlined in the original brochure, are still adhered to, though, with the passage of time, it has become clear that these basic criteria are more useful when taken as guidelines rather than as rules. Common sense and flexibility of approach do much to ensure that Helen House meets families' needs sensitively. For example, although initially it was said that Helen House was intended to cater for children under the age of sixteen, young visitors to Helen House are not suddenly refused help simply because they have reached their sixteenth birthday. Equally, though children are not normally admitted to Helen House for the first time after the age of sixteen, the sensible and sensitive approach to the individual needs of a particular sixteen-year-old and his or her family might well be to admit him or her for terminal or respite care. One thing that *has* changed over the years is that, generally speaking, children coming to Helen House for the first time are iller than first-time visitors in the early days. However, the balance between terminal and respite care admissions remains the same as it has always been, i.e. six beds are for respite care, two for emergency admissions of whatever sort.

Initial enquiries about Helen House and what it might be able to offer a particular child and his or her family might come from the family themselves, or from someone involved with the child in a professional capacity – for example a GP, consultant, social worker or teacher. When dealing with referrals or enquiries, it is necessary to beware of 'worthy third parties'; Helen House would never initiate direct contact with a family on the basis of hearsay. If a 'non-professional' third party makes enquiries on behalf of a child or family, Helen House will send them the brochure and information and suggest that, if it seems appropriate, they ask the family concerned to get in touch themselves. Many telephone calls to Helen House are simply people exploring possibilities and, after a brochure is sent out, no more is heard.

When a family or a professional involved in the care of a child contacts Helen House hoping to refer the child, they are asked to supply a letter from the child's doctor giving full details of his or her condition and needs. Sometimes one of the Helen House doctors might write to the child's doctor following a referral. It has been found to be more constructive if the doctor's letter comes via the family, who are then closely involved from the start with the process which might bring their child to Helen House. If, judging from the information he has of the child from the family and doctor, Roger feels that Helen House can help them and that what the family are looking for is broadly matched by what Helen House can offer them, then he invites the family to come for an interview. However, invitation to attend for interview does not mean a definite commitment by Helen House to help; sometimes, admittedly very rarely, it has been necessary after an interview for the doctors to say, regretfully, that Helen House cannot help a particular family. Sometimes, too, families come for interview, are told that Helen House can help them by offering their child respite care and then go away and make no further contact, or perhaps do not make contact again for several years, until their child is at the end of his or her life. It would seem that for some (admittedly few) families, knowing the 'safety-net' is there is enough.

In this context Roger tells an interesting story. He was contacted a few years ago by a doctor at the John Radcliffe Hospital who told him about a child at the hospital who was terminally ill whom Helen House might be able to help. The family were, understandably, distraught and frightened. The doctor did not feel their needs were being met in hospital, yet they found the idea of taking their gravely ill child home too daunting to consider seriously. Roger visited them at the John Radcliffe Hospital and talked to them at length. He told them that Helen House would like very much to help them and could do so at any time, even immediately. Shortly afterwards, the family, much sustained by Roger's words, took their child home where he died peacefully. They felt immensely relieved that he had died at home, but said they had only felt able to take him home on the strength of their conversation with Roger, because they knew Helen House was there should they fail to cope as they wanted to.

When a family first visits Helen House and comes for interview they are seen by Roger (or Hilary or Ruth) and by a member of the care team. As one of the team puts it, it is less frightening for the family if someone 'non-medical' sits in on the initial interview and also this person can note down the 'human facts' as opposed to the more obviously medical ones which Roger clearly needs to record. The family has a chance to look around the hospice and perhaps meet and talk to other families and children. If, after this initial visit, the family and the Helen House doctors feel that Helen House is appropriate for them and their child, a date for a first stay is arranged. Wherever possible, this first stay involves the whole family, who are encouraged to come with their ill child for a weekend. One thing is felt to be very important in all this and is one reason why a referral from a consultant or doctor or other professional, however detailed the information they supply may be and however appropriate Helen House might seem to be for the child, is not in itself enough to ensure that a child is offered care at Helen House; the family must themselves really want to use the hospice. Talking to families enables Roger and the team member present with him to find out whether families are really happy to come or whether (as occasionally happens) they have felt driven to accept outside help against their inclination by well-meaning relatives or professionals.

On any one shift at Helen House a particular member of the team is in charge of a particular child, doing everything for, and with, that child, whether feeding and washing, talking, playing or taking the child out for walks or on shopping expeditions. All the team at Helen House in the course of their work inevitably meet a large number of different families and will find themselves caring for different children at different times, depending both on their shifts and working hours and on which children happen to be staying at a particular time. Families and children get to know a number of different members of the Helen House team and realize that a child will not always be cared for by the same person. However, every Helen House child and family has at least one 'contact person' on the team, someone who aims to get to know them perhaps a little better than the other team members, who knows their particular circumstances and is aware of any particular problems, difficulties, needs, hopes and fears they may have. The idea behind the 'contact person' system is that in this way you 'avoid people getting lost', to quote a member of the team. The contact person keeps in touch with the child and family between visits to Helen House and aims, by ringing up or writing regularly, to 'keep the lines open'. By keeping in touch in this way, they make it easier for a family to contact the hospice themselves when they need or want to.

There are no rigid rules as to how contact persons are assigned to families. Sometimes the team member who sat in on the family's initial interview with the Medical Director will subsequently become the family's provisional contact person, but not always. Obviously, it makes sense for team members to share particular responsibility for individual children and families fairly evenly, to avoid one team member being so overburdened as to be unable to offer the sort of friendship, reassurance and support the scheme was set up to provide. However, it is also important to remember that children and families will have their own feelings and will perhaps feel drawn to particular members of the team more than to others. This is something the team acknowledge readily. What usually happens when a new family come to Helen House is that the Head Nurse suggests to a team member who perhaps has fewer families of his or her 'own' than other team members at that particular moment, that he or she might like to be the contact person for that family. If mutual confidence and liking develop, that person remains the family's contact person. However, if for any reason at all either the team member or the family do not feel happy with the arrangement then there is a change of contact person. This surely makes sense; we all, after all, choose our friends! One thing I should perhaps say is that families are not necessarily aware that they have a 'contact person' as such; the system is not described to them in such terms. What they do know is that there is a particular person (sometimes more than one person) on the Helen House team who clearly cares about them a great deal. Again, it is the doing, not the describing, that counts.

There are twenty-seven and a half full-time equivalents on

the care team at Helen House. They, with the Administrator, a secretary, the Medical Director and the two other GPs who now support him and an honorary chaplain, make up what could be described as the core staff of Helen House. Helen House also enjoys the loyal support of a number of volunteer helpers. It has never been necessary to advertise for volunteers; when the hospice was still in the planning stage a large number of people got in touch to offer support and help and there has continued to be a steady stream of people coming forward in this way. This stream has usually become a torrent when Helen House has, for some reason, been in the public eye or Sister Frances has, perhaps, appeared on television or spoken on radio. To ensure the smooth running of the system, one of the team is responsible for seeing would-be volunteers, taking on those that are suitable when additional volunteers are needed, and for organizing rotas. Volunteers cannot in any way be seen as unpaid team members; they do not have at all the same duties or responsibilities. Indeed, one of the things that sometimes comes as a disappointment to potential helpers is that volunteers do not work with the children. As the current volunteer's application form puts it, 'The care of the children at Helen House is in the hands of the permanent staff for the sake of continuity.' The role of volunteers and how they are used has evolved over the years since Helen House opened. Initially, when someone expressed an interest in helping at Helen House, he or she was sent an application form to fill in on which, among other things, they underlined on a given list the jobs they were able and willing to undertake. These included cleaning, cooking, gardening, washing-up, ironing, cleaning windows etc. Because things have changed somewhat (for example window-cleaning is now done on contract; ironing is usually done at night by the night staff) volunteers now all, essentially, do the same thing – they help at meal-times, cooking and serving food, clearing up afterwards and tidying the kitchen.

When someone rings or writes to express an interest in

becoming a volunteer, the team member in charge of the volunteers, Marilyn Eyles, sends them an application form to complete, to check their serious intent. When this is returned, a visit is arranged at which Marilyn explains the role of volunteers and shows them round Helen House. She stresses the importance of this 'tour'; it is important to gauge how potential volunteers feel about what goes on at Helen House, how they react to what they see and hear. Some potential volunteers drop out when they realize they will not be closely involved with the very ill children; some clearly have a rather romantic notion of being involved in the more 'picturesque' aspects of what they imagine goes on at Helen House, perhaps seeing themselves exclusively in a soothing, bedside role. Sadly, their idea of what they would do to 'help' in no way accords with the help Helen House actually needs. It is explained to potential volunteers that what is needed is a regular commitment to come in once a week, basically to help over meal-times. There are two volunteers who regularly come in on a Wednesday evening for several hours and cook main meals for the freezer. The other volunteers prepare and serve meals (and do everything that goes with that) on their particular midday or evening slot. By helping in this very practical way, they free the staff on duty to sit at the table with the children and any relatives with them and listen. Meal-times are often the times parents and children talk most freely. The volunteers are themselves invited to join the staff and children at table before serving coffee, loading the dishwasher and clearing up.

Volunteers may not be paid but that does not mean that not much can be expected of them or that, in appointing them, you are less fussy about what you require. As with paid work, it is important to get the right people for the job. As one team member puts it, 'If it's not the right person, it's no help.' People's motives in approaching Helen House in the first place need to be considered. If they are propelled simply by curiosity (or by a burning desire to meet the Duchess of Kent!) they are probably not the right people to help. No more are they the right people if they are looking to Helen House to, in some way, salve their guilt. One potential volunteer helper said recently that she thought she 'ought to help', though she didn't particularly relish the idea, because 'it would be good for me'. Fortunately, Helen House is approached by many enthusiastic, straightforward and kind people who want to help and will do whatever they are told is most helpful, cheerfully and unobtrusively.

Most of the volunteers who help at Helen House are between twenty-five and sixty-five years old. Although there is no hard-and-fast rule, it is felt that twenty-five is a sensible minimum age. Something I find amazing is the distances people are prepared to travel to work as volunteers at Helen House. One volunteer comes regularly on alternate Sundays from Reading; another used to come every Friday from central London until she moved nearer.

A very important member of the 'core staff' at Helen House is the honorary chaplain. Originally we did not envisage there being a chaplain attached to Helen House; although it was recognized that some families might perhaps wish to talk to, or call upon the services of, a minister of religion at some time while their child was staying at Helen House, it was felt that there were ministers locally who would be available and willing to be called upon in such circumstances. However, very soon, the advantages of having one particular person attached to the hospice whom staff and families alike would identify as the person to turn to when the services of a minister were required, became clear. In 1983 the first honorary chaplain, the Reverend Jack Whittaker, was appointed. When he retired the Reverend Michael Smith was appointed as his successor.

Michael (like Jack before him) is not a shadowy, cassocked figure whose presence in Helen House betokens recent or imminent death. The chaplain is very much part of the ongoing life of the hospice; he is someone who is, quite simply, often around, sharing meals, getting to know people and, importantly, letting people get to know him. He approaches children, families and staff as a friend and fellow human being. At the same time, everybody knows they can turn to the chaplain more specifically as a minister, as someone able to fulfil a minister's functions, if they need to.

Over the years the chaplain has, among other things, prayed with families and children, given blessings, organized informal services and conducted funerals, quite apart from simply being with families at times of spiritual need. The chaplain is also very much involved in 'Helen House occasions', such as the annual informal carol service held in the playroom and the yearly reunion for bereaved families. In September 1992 it was Michael Smith who conducted the service of thanksgiving in Christ Church Cathedral, Oxford to mark the tenth anniversary and his predecessor, Jack Whittaker, who led the prayers. Shortly afterwards Michael officiated at the wedding of a member of the Helen House team to the son of another member of the team who himself had worked at Helen House.

Both Jack and Michael became chaplain of Helen House because of their personal qualifications quite as much as their position as ministers of religion. Each of them was, quite simply, the right *person* for the job. Michael has a special affinity with Helen House families because he first came into contact with the hospice in the way they do; his baby son was very ill and Michael and his wife turned to Helen House for help and support. Their beloved son, Jack, died at the hospice at the age of four months.

As was made clear at the outset and is stated in the Helen House brochure, families are welcomed irrespective of race, creed and religion. Helen House exists to meet the requirements of the families who turn to it, to respond to their needs, not to presume to know in advance what those needs might be, whether in the practical or spiritual field. Some families who come do not embrace the Christian faith; others simply have no religious faith of any sort. The fact that there is a chaplain on call and sometimes around the place does not mean that religious activity is on the timetable or that religious feeling is compulsory. The chaplain is there to do what families want of him and he recognizes that this may, sometimes, be nothing at all.

Incidentally, Michael is not at Helen House by any means all the time. He can be called upon when needed and makes a point of coming into the hospice regularly but the work he does there is in addition to his job as vicar of a busy parish.

We have always felt it important that the philosophy and aims of Helen House should be clearly understood and that awareness of the needs of the children and families who turn to the hospice and others in similar situations should be heightened. To this end Sister Frances, the Administrator, members of the Helen House staff and Richard and I continue to give talks when invited and interest in Helen House, whether from professionals or the general public, is encouraged and information forthcoming (where giving such information in no way breaches the privacy of individual children or families). The policy at Helen House is one of openness, provided this does not conflict with peace and privacy for those who use the hospice. For obvious reasons, it is not possible for the general public or indeed professionals not directly involved with the children to be shown round Helen House as a matter of course, but there are now regular open afternoons for professionals once a month which anyone interested can attend by arrangement. We realize that what Helen House provides is only part of the spectrum of support and provision which is (or should be) available to children with life-threatening illness and their families and feel it is important that those involved with other aspects of care and types of provision should understand what Helen House aims to do, just as Helen House should understand their aims. Communication is very important if care and provision are to be enhanced.

As well as the policy of openness Helen House has chosen to adopt, there is the openness that is, quite rightly, forced upon the hospice – the openness to inspection. Helen House is registered with Oxfordshire Health Authority as a nursing

A House Called Helen

home, which involves paying an annual fee based on the number of beds and being subject to regular twice-yearly inspections. One of these is a 'notified inspection' but the other can take place at any time, without warning. Anything and everything comes under the scrutiny of the Nursing Home Registration and Monitoring Officer – nursing practices, safety, hygiene, care of drugs, disposal of waste, dangerous drugs and sharps, menus. Bad, and sometimes sensational, publicity about standards of provision and care in nursing homes of all sorts over the last few years has led Health Authorities (even those that were already very thorough and conscientious) to tighten up on their checks and inspections. Helen House is also inspected regularly by the Fire Officer, who reports to the Nursing Home Registration Monitoring Officer, and by the inspector authorized by the Oxfordshire Health Authority under the Registered Homes Act 1984 (previously the area Pharmacist) and of course could receive visits of inspection from other official bodies – the Health and Safety Executive, for example, or the Charity Commissioners.

While everyone accepts that regulations are in force to protect and safeguard organizations and individuals, on occasion they can, in their application, lead to misunderstandings. This happened recently in the case of Helen House. Helen House is registered as having eight beds for very ill children. On a recent visit, following a conversation with the Head Nurse, the Nursing Home Registration and Monitoring Officer realized that it was possible that on occasion there just might be more than eight very ill children at Helen House; this might happen if, for example, a family arrived with their child in the morning and the child vacating the room this newly-arrived child was to occupy was not being taken home until the afternoon. Having on the premises (albeit very temporarily) more than the number of ill children they were registered to care for could put Helen House in a difficult position from the legal and insurance point of view were anything, by any chance, to go wrong. To get round this difficulty, the Nursing

178

Home Registration and Monitoring Officer said that Helen House should register as a provider of two day-care places for very ill children. When it was stated in the local press that Helen House had recently been granted two day-care places, many people reading this imagined that Helen House was expanding and departing from its original plan. Misunderstandings like this are often hard to dispel.

What is more, the strict application of increasingly rigorous safety regulations puts a heavy financial burden on organizations, which, in the case of small concerns, can be crippling. Helen House is fortunate in that people continue to give generously to support its aims but, nevertheless, it is hard to see funds donated by people anxious to help Helen House in its work having to be spent on such things as yet larger illuminated exit signs – particularly when the previous ones were approved only a year before! Moreover, it becomes increasingly difficult, as safety and fire regulations are applied across the board and often with little regard to significant differences in scale and circumstances, for a place like Helen House, which aims to provide care in a setting as much like a family home as possible, to remain homely and 'intimate'.

I am often asked whether Helen House provides counselling for the families who use, or have used, the hospice. Counselling was never in our remit. Helen House was set up to be a home-from-home for very ill children and to offer support and friendship to them and their families. True friendship involves a balance between giving and taking and flourishes when it is rooted in equality. The members of the team at Helen House offer friendship to ill children and their families by coming alongside them in their pain and grief; they do not claim to advise them, or, however subtly, to influence or modify their behaviour or feelings by virtue of professionally-acquired skills.

However, in saying that Helen House does not offer counselling, we run up against a problem of terminology, against the fact that the word counselling is currently a very overworked word which, increasingly, in its modern usage, is coming to replace 'conversation', 'chatting', 'discussion', plenty of which goes on at Helen House. Good professional counselling requires a particular aptitude and thorough training in addition, of course, to specialist knowledge of the particular field in which you operate. We live in a world where the pace of change is accelerating, and where, too, increasingly, the changes that are taking place leave few of us unaffected, and indeed can demand a radical overhaul of attitudes and life-style. This can be deeply unsettling. In such a climate it is perhaps not surprising that more and more people are turning to counsellors for help, whether in their professional or private lives. Counsellors are in great demand.

However, side by side with this growth in often highly-specialized counselling, there is a growing tendency to use the word 'counselling' very loosely, to use it to describe any meaningful conversation in which one person even half listens to another. Given the number of times that the word 'counselling' replaces the words 'talk' or 'conversation', you could be excused for thinking that the exchange of ideas between individuals on an equal footing was a thing of the past! Perhaps this is further evidence of a crisis of confidence in our society, another example of how human qualities are undervalued unless they are labelled with some professional term. We need constantly to reaffirm the value and validity of human impulses, instincts and values. We must beware of humanity being hijacked.

Counselling may not be offered at Helen House, but opportunities to talk abound. Parents, children, members of the team and friends talk about anything and everything. Seemingly light-hearted conversations can develop into deep discussions; equally, deep discussions can suddenly dissolve into light-hearted anecdote. Discussions can involve quite a lot of people (around the supper table for instance) or can be between just two people. Conversations are not timetabled or planned. Often some of the most deep and far-reaching discussions take place in the most 'domestic' situations – over the washing-up or while weeding in the garden, for example. It is a sign of feeling at ease, of feeling you are among friends, when you are able to bring up whatever is uppermost in your mind wherever and whenever you feel inclined. One mother once told me what a relief she found it to come to Helen House because there her seemingly inconsequential leaps in conversation from the anecdotal (and even trivial) to the profound (and often deeply upsetting) was not seen as strange or something she should be helped to overcome. 'It's wonderful here', she said. 'Nobody thinks you're mad.'

Soon after Helen House opened, a concerned (and trained) individual who was anxious to help was very eager to provide bereavement counselling for families. She offered her services between certain hours one day a week. This simply did not work, for a number of fairly predictable reasons. Families who might perhaps have benefited from such counselling often were not staying at Helen House at the appointed time and lived too far away to come in specially. Moreover, the really black times bereaved relatives went through, the times they felt the greatest need to talk, often simply did not coincide with the allotted counselling hours. Grief is unpredictable and does not operate to a timetable.

A second attempt to have some sort of forum for discussion and sharing of feelings proved a little more successful. This was the initiative of the mother of a young boy who died a year before Helen House opened. She felt that she and others like her would find it enormously helpful to meet and talk about their feelings, and for a time she organized regular evening meetings in the discussion room at Helen House. These drew together a number of parents (mostly mothers) who came both to give and to receive comfort. The meetings fizzled out after about two years because the mother who was the driving force behind them found that the demands of her growing family (growing in terms of number as well as of age!) made it impossible for her to continue in her active role with the bereavement group.

181

A House Called Helen

An initiative which has proved extremely successful more recently is bereavement visiting. This was really the idea of Tessa Wilkinson, a Montessori-trained nursery school teacher who originally came to Helen House as a volunteer. Tessa was initially the only volunteer working at Helen House. One of her first tasks was to sort through the three-hundred-odd letters which had arrived at the hospice even before it opened from people wanting to offer their services and from these to identify further volunteers. (Tessa, in fact, 'ran' the volunteers for four years.) After six months as a volunteer Tessa joined the Helen House team. Working on the team and getting to know individual children and their families well, she was struck by a recurrent theme in these families' accounts of their life at home with a very ill child and later when that child died. Most of them spoke, in one way or another, of their feelings of isolation and of the loneliness that engulfed them as they battled with the huge physical and emotional burden they had to bear. These feelings were not miraculously dissipated when their child died, in fact the feelings of loneliness usually then became even more acute.

Tessa became convinced that there was a role here for a bereavement visitor, a specific person to work with bereaved families, someone who would go into the family home as a friend from Helen House. (This person would be in addition to the family's 'contact person'.) Looking back, Tessa says: 'The need seemed to be for someone to visit, and to *keep* visiting the families during the dark months or years following the death of their child.' In a sense, the job of a bereavement visitor would involve a continuation (with differences) of the philosophy of Helen House. It would involve coming alongside bereaved families as a friend, reducing their feelings of isolation and seeking to reassure them.

Tessa herself was the first (and, initially, only) Helen House bereavement visitor. She remained a member of the team and in fact worked on the team at Helen House for one day a week. The rest of the time she spent visiting bereaved families. When her husband's work took the family to Coventry and Tessa

182

could no longer get to Helen House easily and often, she had to give up working on the Helen House team and took instead to bereavement visiting almost full-time. Interestingly, bereavement visiting without direct input from Helen House through working shifts worked less well; to take the philosophy of Helen House out into individual homes clearly required continuing full contact with Helen House and all that went on there. Although Tessa continued to come to Helen House regularly once a week, she no longer had the close contact with families and the care team that actually working shifts at the hospice had previously brought her.

As her work-load increased, Tessa was joined in her bereavement visiting work by another member of the Helen House team, Sarah Tiptaft. The work of bereavement visiting was now taking up one and a half full-time posts. When Tessa decided, upon her husband's taking up his new post as Bishop's Chaplain in Guildford, that she could no longer continue working for Helen House, her place as a bereavement visitor was taken by Rod Sharp who had been working on the team at Helen House for about seven years. When Sarah (now Mrs Sarah Barrell) left in 1992 to have a baby, she was replaced as a bereavement visitor by Bronwen Bennett. Interestingly, my first meeting with Bronwen had been when she came to visit us in our home in the first year of Helen's illness bringing us much comfort.

Rod and Bronwen are based at Helen House. They each work at least one day a week on the team, which they see as an essential way of keeping in touch and remaining attuned to the philosophy of Helen House. The rest of their time is spent visiting Helen House families up and down the country. They make sure that they discuss their work and exchange ideas regularly (they see it as particularly important that there should be close communication with the family's contact person) and they keep diaries with brief records of their visits and activities, as Tessa had done before them. These they discuss with the Head Nurse from time to time and in addition they have regular meetings at Helen House with Helen Woolley. Helen Woolley's is a supportive role and the bereavement visitors say she is a useful sounding-board for new ideas they may have about their work.

When a child dies there is not just one bereavement; in addition to the immeasurable pain of losing their child, the family also suffers the loss of all sorts of other friends and sources of professional support. Rod and Bronwen see bereavement visiting as a way of making sure that families know they do not have to lose the friendship and support of Helen House because they have lost their child (the child they perhaps saw as their passport to that friendship and support). They offer parents the choice of making a break or continuing contact. Choice remains with the family and this is seen as crucial. If a family opts for continuing contact the pattern of visits is mutually agreed by them and the bereavement visitors. For the sake of convenience, at the end of a visit the bereavement visitor will almost always agree with the family a time and date for a further visit, but the family can postpone or cancel this at any time if they so wish. The important thing is that the initiative comes from the family because they know best what helps them.

Often Rod or Bronwen will visit families who live a considerable distance from Oxford, which can mean spending a night away from home. However, neither of them stays the night with the family they are visiting. As Rod puts it, 'An open-ended visit can be counter-productive.' As bereavement visitors, they need to remember that there is a specific reason for their being with the families and their role is to focus on the families' needs without putting any additional pressure on them. However, while their role is perhaps more clearly laid down than that of a close friend, it is by no means hedged about by arbitrary rules and restrictions. Rod was once talking about his work to a friend who is a professional counsellor. He talked of a conversation he had had with a family over tea at their house. His counsellor friend expostulated: 'Oh, I'd never *eat* with a family!' and went on to explain that this would erode the vital barrier that must exist between a counsellor and his 'client'. The relationship between Helen House bereavement visitors and the families they visit is a much less formal one than that between a counsellor and his client. The friendship component is much stronger. Both Rod and Bronwen feel it is vital, if they are to help the families they visit in the Helen House spirit, that they do not deny the two-way nature of the relationship or establish, albeit unwittingly, a 'them and us' situation.

Although they and other members of the team who sometimes visit bereaved families must always remember that there is a specific reason for their visiting a family, namely to support and help them, how the bereavement visitors do that will be determined by what the family wants or needs on that particular occasion. Sometimes a visit is spent looking through the family photo album and listening to reminiscences, sometimes it is spent helping the family make specific plans – for a holiday, or a memorial service, perhaps – and sometimes a visit involves going out with a family, perhaps to visit their child's grave or perhaps to help them get over the hurdle of going to the supermarket or some similarly public place for the first time since their child died. Sometimes a visit is spent providing practical information, for example about organizations that might be able to help with particular problems or difficulties. Rod stresses the importance of seeing Helen House as not exclusive and the need to encourage families to make use of other organizations where appropriate – The Compassionate Friends, or Cruse, for example.

Inevitably, as the years pass, the work-load of bereavement visitors from Helen House may well grow as more children who have stayed at Helen House die. Whether it will be necessary to have more than two bereavement visitors in the future is difficult to say; it will depend on whether families opt for continuing contact with Helen House after their child has died and, if they do, for how long they wish that contact to continue. As always, it will be the families whose needs will determine the service; it will not be a case of families' needs being massaged to fit in to the existing service.

Once a year, usually in November, around the time of Helen House's birthday, when the hospice is closed for a week, what is known as the bereavement weekend takes place. This gives Helen House families whose ill child has died a chance to return to Helen House if they so wish, to meet all the staff again and also other families, some of whom they may have got to know quite well and, in a short service, to remember their children who have died. Many families find it hard (however much they may want to) to return to Helen House during the 'working year' and the bereavement weekend gives them a specific opportunity, a valid reason for coming back. Moreover, fresh contact (initiated by Helen House) makes it easier for families to establish regular contact again (possibly after quite a long break) if they so wish.

The families who come to Helen House almost invariably comment on the garden and its peace and beauty. As you look out from the windows of Helen House across the garden you see beyond it the beautiful mature trees in the convent garden (including a huge copper beech whose lofty majesty Frances compares to that of a cathedral and under which she and Helen would sometimes sit together when Helen was staying with her) and beyond them the outline of the convent chapel. The bell ringing to call the sisters to prayer is a familiar sound to everyone at Helen House. Although none of the sisters from All Saints Convent are at present on the staff, they all support Helen House through their prayers and take a keen interest in all that goes on at the hospice, which remains under the umbrella of the Society of All Saints. Without the sisters' initial support for Frances's pioneering venture, Helen House would never have come into being and the staff of the hospice feel sustained by the continuing support of 'their friends across the garden'.

Helen House is incorporated in the Society of All Saints. The individuals who run the hospice are answerable to Mother Helen, the Reverend Mother Superior General of the Society of All Saints. In theory, the Society of All Saints could, if they wished, elect to take over the day-to-day running of Helen House; in practice, they delegate this to the Administrator and Head Nurse. The Helen House accounts are presented to the Trustees of the Society of All Saints at their regular twice-yearly meetings which the Administrator and Head Nurse always attend in order to give a full report on, and answer questions about, the work of Helen House. The Helen House accounts are open to inspection on request but are not published in an annual report and (as was agreed from the start) the Helen House newsletters never contain direct appeals for funds.

Helen House is still funded entirely by voluntary donations; it is completely independent of state funding. No family pays any fee when their child stays at the hospice. As well as the steady income it gets from covenants and legacies, Helen House also continues to receive money raised by individuals, schools and organizations of all sorts by their fund-raising activities. Before Helen House opened, when there was a tremendous flurry of fund-raising activity in aid of the hospice, we were warned that enthusiasm and fund-raising zeal might evaporate once Helen House was up and running; often a charity is hugely in favour for a time but then supplanted in the public interest by a different good cause. To our delight, Helen House has confounded these predictions; although there was a drop in the number of activities organized on behalf of the hospice once its building costs had been met and the hospice was actually operational, this drop was never of the dramatic kind we were warned to expect and Helen House has remained a cause that many people clearly still wish to support. Fund-raising continues and for this we are enormously grateful.

Inevitably, the cost of running Helen House is rising all the time; not only do staff salaries rise in accordance with rises in nurses' pay but basic overheads are increasing all the time. The telephone bill, fairly predictably, is high and likely to rise if the number of families using Helen House or in contact with the hospice increases. Families staying with their ill children at Helen House often need to telephone other relatives, often in distant parts of the country, and of course the staff at the hospice keep in touch with families by telephone. Telephone conversations of this kind cannot always be brief and businesslike.

Helen House is fortunate in that it has been successful in attracting interest and support and this interest and support has been sustained. However, success can in itself bring problems, some of which might be described as more irritating than fundamental while others could necessitate thorough re-appraisal of aims and approach. Coping with success is not always easy. Helen House is generally considered to be very successful and is a 'first' in the field of care of children with life-threatening illness, an emotive field and one where emotion can so easily degenerate into sentimentality. This combination has made the hospice the victim of media hype and made it hard at times to keep clearly before everybody two fundamentally important things; first, Helen House is a modest venture and, second, what it does is very simple. This message is sometimes swamped in the hype surrounding the hospice and there is the danger that the very simple philosophy and straightforward aims of Helen House will be distorted in the glossy (and often sentimental) telling. It does seem, too, that people are now so attuned to glamour and sophistication that they find it impossible to accept that something simple and uncomplicated could be radiantly successful.

In general terms, success can make you feel you know all the answers, it can make you stop thinking about what you are doing and make you complacent. In the case of Helen House, if they were lulled into complacency by the apparent success of the hospice, team members could soon cease to be receptive to the views and feelings of those around them. They could soon find that they had stopped listening to the children and families they wanted to help. Soon theories rather than the varying needs of individuals would be determining their behaviour. When, in the early days of Helen's illness, Frances helped us by sometimes looking after Helen, she did so as a friend who wanted to help us in whatever way we found most useful; she did not approach us because she had a number of theories on the care of very ill children that she wished to test. The staff at Helen House are mindful of this and of how success could, if they were not careful, make them approach the individual through the general and not the other way round. As one member of the team puts it: 'You have to listen to families and children with your whole being. The day you say "Helen House does this" you have established a new set of theories and theories are what we were trying to escape from in the first place with Helen House.' The fact that there was no blueprint for Helen House was, she feels, in this respect 'our salvation'.

Perhaps the most serious problem success has brought to Helen House stems from the fact that more and more families are now contacting the hospice and making enquiries, in particular about respite care. A few years ago, with pressure on the hospice growing, it became necessary to look again at admissions policy and at the impact any change in approach here might have on the quality of the care and support offered.

Basically, there are two ways of looking at respite care. You can say, quite simply, that 'all comers' are welcomed and accommodated if there is a free bed on the particular day or night in question. Alternatively, you can decide to take on your books only a certain number of families, in order not to find yourself, as you take on more and more families, having to say no increasingly often to those asking for respite care. Basically, it is a choice between offering something (probably respite care very occasionally and in a somewhat impersonal way) to a relatively large number of families and offering something more sustained (regular respite care, support and developing friendship) to a smaller number and, sadly, nothing to some would-be users of the hospice.

However, these seemingly clear-cut options were not what the Medical Director and Head Nurse had before them a few years ago when growing unease and anxiety generated by increasing demands on the hospice led them to think hard about their approach to admissions. Helen House had started out with the idea that the quality of what it offered was very important. Staff, it was felt, needed to get to know families and to build up a relationship in order to offer real support based on knowledge, understanding, and empathy. In making the decision as to whether to maintain a limit on the number of families on the list of those using Helen House, the Head Nurse and the Medical Director (and all involved in the discussions) had to remember that they were not starting from scratch; there was a large number of families already coming to Helen House who had grown to depend on the quality of care and the real friendship the hospice offered them. Taking on more families and going down the path, essentially, of saying that an empty bed even for one night is inexcusable if there is a family somewhere (even one the hospice staff do not know at all) whose child could use it, would mean pulling the carpet out from under the feet of those families already using the hospice, suddenly withdrawing from them what they had come to depend on. When planning from scratch you can, perhaps, argue strongly for spreading care thinly to go round more people and concerning yourself perhaps slightly less with quality (even though this was *never* Helen House's stance). However, when you are considering changing to this approach from a policy of concentrating care on a rather smaller (but never exclusive in absolute terms) number, you have to consider the effects of the change on those who have benefited from, and come to depend on, what you have offered to date.

After much deliberation it was decided that it did not make sense for Helen House to accept on to its books every family that turned to the hospice for help. The quality-of-care argument won the day over the numbers argument. Families would only be taken on if it was felt that Helen House could

offer them something ongoing, sustained and personal in terms
of care. In this the hospice was continuing to operate essentially
as envisaged in the planning days, i.e. it really was offering
support and friendship to children and their families. After all,
friendship in any meaningful sense only develops where there
is close acquaintance and familiarity and is not withdrawn
when not convenient, and support is truly helpful and
reassuring only when you can depend on it. Also, an aim of
the hospice has always been to 'stay alongside' families going
through the anguish of seeing a much-loved child become very
ill, deteriorate and die. There is a limit to the number of families
you can 'stay alongside' in any meaningful sense.

There are no precise limits on the number of families Helen
House is prepared to have on its books at any one time. The
demands different children and families make on the hospice
vary enormously, which makes planning based purely on
numbers rather foolish. However, it is felt that the hospice
ceases to be able to function to the hoped-for standard when
the number of families rises above *roughly* one hundred, and
this number provides a useful guideline. One thing that must
be made clear, however, is that terminal care is always offered
when requested.

Commenting on the apparent success of Helen House, people
have on several occasions asked us why Helen House does not
expand to accommodate more children. The temptation to see
the success of a venture as a reason for expansion is great, but
the dangers involved in expansion are correspondingly great.
By enlarging something you do not necessarily get more of the
same; you get something that is qualitatively different.
Expansion should be viewed with caution; you should never
overlook the fact that perhaps the success of your enterprise
stems directly from its small size, clear remit and modest aims.
In the case of Helen House, families come (and return) for the
very reason that the hospice is small and intimate. Small would
certainly appear to be beautiful.

Whether this is so and whether Helen House is successful

is best gauged by asking the families and children who use the hospice how it has helped them. It is impossible to elicit the views of all the children who come to stay at Helen House because many of them, sadly, cannot speak or are too ill to say very much. However, spontaneous comments made by a number of children over the years suggest that children are happy and relaxed at Helen House and enjoy coming. Comments on seemingly trivial or insignificant things are perhaps more revealing about what they like about the atmosphere than might at first appear. 'I like making cakes when I want to', shows that not only are children able to indulge in favourite hobbies and be active (and messy!) but that there is no timetable or 'right time' laid down for activities. The absence of rules and a timetable at Helen House and the way personal tastes are indulged is also apparent from such remarks as: 'You can have breakfast in bed if you want to'; 'It's like a hotel'; 'I like going in the jacuzzi when I feel like it'. The fact that even children as ill as the children Helen House caters for appreciate stimulation and activity is clear from such remarks as: 'I'm never bored here'; 'You can have fun with the staff'; 'They have time for you'.

Perhaps the greatest tribute of all to the team at Helen House and the most positive proof we have of the way in which the hospice actually *does* seem like a family home to the children who come for respite care, is provided by a question put by a child to one of the team one day over lunch. 'Rod,' he asked, 'when do you go to work?'

For the parents and relatives who care for very ill children at home (often over a very long period of time) bringing their children to Helen House is often a huge relief, simply in terms of the way it eases their physical burden. One mother of a young girl said that with her daughter lovingly cared for by the staff downstairs, she was able to go up to the parents' flat and have her first night of uninterrupted sleep for twelve years. Later, like other parents and families, she felt able to go away with an easy mind and leave her daughter to be cared for while she and her husband took a holiday. Many parents comment on how they feel able, perhaps for the first time in their child's illness, to leave him or her, because they are confident that at Helen House all the little things that their child finds helpful, soothing or reassuring will be done for him or her. 'The staff have time for you'; 'Nothing is too much trouble'; and – something that is like balm to the battered souls of many Helen House parents whose child's condition inevitably imposes all sorts of restrictions upon them and puts them in great need of the goodwill and support of those around them – 'At Helen House you never feel you're a nuisance.'

Many of the parents and relatives I have spoken to over the years comment on the peace and beauty of Helen House. 'I never thought it would be so beautiful', one parent said to me, commenting on her child's bedroom and the view from the window. Nearly all the parents comment on the garden, its beauty and tranquillity and the pleasure their well children find playing in it.

Feeling surrounded by love and concern is very sustaining to the families who come to Helen House – often with great apprehension at first and not knowing quite what to expect. Several families have spoken of their reluctance initially to turn to Helen House for help because they felt that by doing so they were 'admitting there was no hope'. When they did eventually overcome that reluctance, the relief was enormous. The parents of a little boy who died at Helen House from a brain tumour subsequently wrote an open letter to other parents who might resist the idea of turning to a hospice, seeing it, as they had once done, as 'a place of no hope'. Describing their experiences when they first brought their son Martin home from hospital, they wrote:

> We refused to give up hope that he might live, and avoided visiting Helen House, though several people had suggested that we could be helped there. Eventually, when we were tired and desperate and

Martin was too ill to stay at home any longer, we came to look.

As soon as we saw the bright new building, the cheerful faces, the beautiful furnishings and tempting toys, we knew that here was a place where Martin would be well cared for, our elder son would have fun and we would have a rest. It soon felt as if the staff shared our problems, and it lightened our burden during the final weeks of Martin's life. If there is any hope for sick children, it is here.

The relief parents feel when they come to Helen House is not just the relief they naturally feel at an easing of their physical load; interestingly, many parents speak as much of the emotional relief as of the physical relief they find at the hospice. It is a relief to be able to 'lean a bit', to 'drop pretences', to feel that 'your feelings are accepted whatever they are', 'the staff are never shocked'. Most important of all, parents speak of the way the staff make them feel their child is special and, in spite of everything, a *person*.

A basic fear of the unknown will always mean that death is something that many people are afraid of. The fact that death has been so effectively removed from the field of human experience and placed increasingly in a medical setting, makes it even more remote and mysterious and not something over the circumstances of which we have much control. For the parents of a child with a life-threatening illness there are additional sources of pain and anxiety. They feel isolated, victims of the acute embarrassment many people feel at the death, or approaching death, of a child; such a death is, after all, so unnatural. Connected with this, is the overwhelming grief they feel at seeing the child they gave birth to, their link with the future, die.

In addition to the widespread fear of death generally that many people harbour, the parents of a child with a life-threatening illness feel very apprehensive about how they will cope emotionally when their child dies and, more specifically, about how death happens, what it is like. Bringing their children to Helen House for respite care, many parents of very ill children have found that their fear and apprehension have been greatly reduced by being at the hospice when another child has died, by seeing how the death of a child can be, in a sense, incorporated into life. One family speaks of their experience here in very positive terms. The parents were on one of their first visits to Helen House and had chosen to stay with their child. A young boy staying with his parents was clearly very ill and near the end of his life. However, he was in no distress or discomfort and was quite peaceful and his parents felt it would be nice for him to be fully part of things, so they wheeled him on his bed down to the playroom to be with other children and members of the team. The day was a very happy one of conversation, play, music and laughter. At the end of the day, the very ill boy was prepared for the night as usual. He died in his mother's arms. The couple telling this story say how much it helped them to have been around in Helen House that day, how their fear of death was dispelled by their realization that death is not necessarily something to which you progress through increasing isolation from, and insulation against, life. Explaining what had helped them, they said of the child that had died, 'You see, he was in the midst of life right up to the very end.'

Many of the aspects of Helen House that families speak of most positively are those very features we felt to be important in the planning stage. Reflecting on this, the Administrator commented recently that it was amazing how much we appeared to have got right when planning Helen House. Certainly, in the years since the hospice opened there has been no need to make fundamental changes in approach. The basic philosophy remains the same and in terms of practical provision and day-to-day management any modifications have been of the 'fine-tuning' variety only. The closeness of Helen House today to the original plan is clear.

A House Called Helen

I do not find this as surprising as some people clearly do. If we have got it right this is probably because, in planning help and support for very ill children and their families, we had a much-loved ill child living at home and a family with clear needs, both practical and emotional, (and experience of how the existing 'caring services' failed to address those needs directly) as a model. Helen House sprang from a close connection with actual need, not from an abstract study of possible requirements. From the start, it was trying to do something on a small scale, which made it easier to put children and families first. What Helen House is trying to achieve was at the outset, and is still today, defined in a specific and limited way.

'We are small enough to know what we are saying,' one of the team remarked recently. An important corollary of this (and something that I hope will never change) is that Helen House makes no claims beyond its own experience and knowledge (although some would make them for us!). The minute you start making claims beyond your competence and knowledge you risk jeopardizing the purity, and indeed effectiveness and success, of your venture. What Helen House offers is based on the familiar, the known, tempered by humility about the unknown.

'I can only speak for myself' – long may this be the motto of Helen House; but where Helen House speaks for itself may it do so with confidence.

196

8

Reflections on Years of Caring

In one sense, but one sense only, the story of Helen House is complete at this point. How the hospice came into existence and what it does has been set out and the philosophy that sustains it adumbrated. But of course Helen House does not operate in a vacuum and the climate in which it functions is important. This climate inevitably influences, and even, to some extent, shapes, the hospice's role. The continuing story of Helen House lies in the way it carries on responding to the needs of the families who come to it for help and these are inevitably affected by the difficulties, problems and attitudes the families encounter in the wider context, by the prevailing climate in society.

For those involved in the work of Helen House and indeed those who might seek to extend or perhaps emulate its work, it is, therefore, useful to have some understanding and awareness of what the families they seek to help may experience in their day-to-day life outside the hospice. Their ability to help and support effectively is nourished and sustained by such an awareness and understanding.

It is for this reason that I decided to describe in this chapter some of the experiences we have had caring for Helen at home over the years and to touch on our feelings about them and about some of the prevailing attitudes and approaches within society and some of the terminology now in use. From conversations with many families in broadly similar circumstances to ours I can say with confidence that although the experiences and feelings are personal they are by no means untypical.

*   *   *

A House Called Helen

It is now more than fourteen years since we brought Helen out of hospital to be at home with us where she belonged. Although we have never really thought of ourselves in such terms, we have been for those fourteen years, and remain today, 'carers'. The term 'carer' is now so widely used and generally understood that it is hard to believe that when we first took Helen out of hospital the word was not in common use. Perhaps, though, even if it had been we still would not have thought of ourselves as 'carers', any more than we do now. We love and care for Helen in all her helplessness just as we love and care for our two other daughters, even if, of course, their needs are very different from hers, being those of independent, active, healthy young girls. Somehow, to put a formal label on our role in relation to our beloved Helen strips what we do for her of its naturalness and, in a sense, suggests a formal appointment to the job of doing what we instinctively *want* to do.

I realize that the fact that I (and others in similar situations, too, I am sure) feel this way can bring us all enormous problems. Many partners, parents, offspring and other relatives devotedly look after very ill, helpless or disabled loved ones with little or no support or help of any kind. Because they see this caring as a natural outcome of their relationship to, or love for, the person they care for, their hard work is taken for granted; it is assumed that what they do willingly they do effortlessly and can do unaided. We hear quite a lot about the poverty trap, but less about what I would call 'the love trap'. Perhaps we must accept the label 'carer', however inappropriate it feels, simply in order to get help.

Over the last fourteen years we have learnt much about the problems of long-term care and also, more specifically, about the pain and loneliness of having a very ill or helpless child. Leaving aside possible financial worries, the difficulties and problems facing anyone looking after a very ill or disabled person divide, very roughly, into two categories, the practical (carrying the physical burden and getting the support and information you need) and the emotional (coping with your feelings and the feelings and attitudes of other people). Of course, problems in the first category can make dealing with problems in the second category much harder and vice versa. Battling with physical problems (lifting and carrying, struggling to bath a helpless person unaided, or to transport them to a hospital appointment single-handed) can make you very tired and therefore much more fragile emotionally and can exacerbate feelings of isolation and unhappiness. Equally, if you are feeling emotionally drained (as we always feel after Helen's birthday, for example) it is difficult to summon up the energy to carry on with the physical tasks that need to be done – and done again and again.

We had a foretaste of the problems relating to information while Helen was still in hospital. We had no idea of what help or support might be available to us if and when we eventually were able to take Helen home with us. We found it difficult to make firm plans for a future we found it painful to think about and which was, in any case, so uncertain. However, a young doctor suggested to us one day that we might be eligible for an attendance allowance, a Social Security benefit for those looking after the severely ill and disabled. We mentioned this to the hospital social worker on one of the frequent occasions when she 'dropped by for a chat' as we sat by Helen's bed. She had just about heard of the allowance but had no information about it. By chance Richard remembered having seen an article about Social Security benefits in *Which?*, the magazine of the Consumers' Association of which we were members. He managed to turn up the article and we read it carefully. It transpired that, to be sure of drawing this benefit in respect of Helen as soon as we brought her home, we had to claim within four months of the onset of her disability. It was now very nearly four months since Helen had been left helpless following her operation, so we needed to act fast. We managed to get hold of the relevant forms and fill them in and fortunately when, after six months in hospital, we took Helen home, we received the attendance allowance to which we were entitled.

Thus we learnt while Helen was still in hospital what was to be confirmed on repeated occasions subsequently – that the burden was on us to find out about what we were entitled to, that some professionals were happy to 'chat things over' but rarely came forward with practical help or information. We gave a copy of the *Which?* article to the hospital social worker in the hope that she might be able to provide information to other families who were probably missing out on what was their right.

That the professionals themselves often know little about the benefits and services available to the ill and disabled people under their care is clear from a programme on the Children Act broadcast on Radio 4 in 1991. One of the people interviewed on this programme was the mother of an autistic child, who also happened to be a doctor. Her experience puts the problem in stark perspective; she said that not even as an informed GP did she know what help was available to her child and her family and that nobody made much of an effort to tell her. She said: 'We were left out right at the beginning and we did not receive any help. We missed out on an attendance allowance. We did not have that until Richard was seven and we could have had that from when he was two. We had never heard of respite care.' At the end of her interview the GP expressed the hope that the obligation that, under the Children Act, will now be on the local authority to give the information out, will help, though she was not confident that with the resources available the information would percolate down. 'I think it very likely that there will not be the funds to advise everybody.'

Talking to families from all over the country at Helen House, I realize that there is a very wide variation in the amount and quality of information different families receive in different parts of the country and, as a result, in the help they get. Services and provision are patchy. Yet surely something as important as this should not be left so much to chance or be so dependent on the persistence and drive of the carers? Carers have enough to cope with; the caring professions (if they are to be worthy of that name) should sometimes reach out to the carers, not leave them always to take the initiative.

Knowing where you should be able to get information is the first hurdle; extracting it is the next. I, like many other people I have spoken to, have often seen my efforts in this direction come to nought. A recent example was when I filled in a form on the back of a booklet about benefits for the disabled that I had picked up in the local Post Office. The form was a request for further information on which you ticked the useful information leaflets you would like to receive. I duly sent off the form but received nothing. On several occasions forms completed according to instructions have failed to elicit the promised response and it is surprising how many letters go unacknowledged and unanswered.

Once you have the information, getting what this information tells you you are entitled to is the next problem. We experienced this early on with the distressing saga of Helen's wheelchair and since then have been shocked to realize the extent to which the time and hard work a carer can (or cannot) put in determines the benefits, basic support and services they and the disabled, ill or elderly person they care for receive (or do not receive). People who are already hugely burdened and emotionally drained should not have to fight in this way for basic provision. Struggles and battles are exhausting and something you really do not have time for. Moreover, if what you are (or, in cases like ours, your ill child is) entitled to is given seemingly only grudgingly and certainly with great delay and only after great persistence on your part, you begin to feel that you are over-demanding, you feel guilty about always asking (even if it is often for the same one thing, again and again) and you feel extremely demoralized at being cast in the role of strident, assertive, troublesome 'taker'. How far removed from reality this is; most people looking after a

201

helpless, disabled or very ill partner, relative or friend are givers, endlessly giving love, time and energy and if they are demanding, this is only in terms of what they ask their bodies to do in support of what their minds and hearts tell them is needed. The only 'taking' most carers know about is in the context of the toll their exhausting lifestyle takes on their health and other relationships.

This lifestyle is made all the more exhausting by the fact that it is impossible to rely on those whose responsibility it is to provide certain basic services and support, to do so. We have had ample experience of this. One particularly distressing instance related to educational provision for Helen. Since she has been of school age Helen has attended the special unit for profoundly multiply-handicapped children at a !ocal special school. We cannot speak highly enough of the staff who over the years have worked with Helen; they have all, without exception, been caring, imaginative and unstinting in their efforts to do everything possible to enhance the lives of the children in their care. Sadly, however, the attitude of our Local Education Authority and Health Authority to children with special needs has not always been positive and indeed the authorities have shown the greatest reluctance to fulfil their obligations under the 1981 Education Act. The recent report by the Audit Commission (*Getting in on the Act* 1992) reveals that this dereliction of duty on the part of Local Education Authorities and Health Authorities is to be found country-wide.

We came up against the authorities' apparent lack of concern about their responsibilities under the 1981 Education Act and, indeed, their obstructive attitude, in relation to the recognition of Helen's special needs. All children with special needs are supposed to have a multi-professional assessment and on the basis of the reports drawn up by the professionals who assess the child (these might include doctors, speech therapists, physiotherapists, educational psychologists and teachers) a detailed statement of the child's needs is drawn up and it is then the duty of the Local Education and Health Authorities to make appropriate provision to ensure that these needs are met. Like many other parents we were, for years, unaware of this procedure and how the system operated and nobody sought to tell us about it. It was not until Helen was approaching her teens (at which time a child's statement comes up for review and, if necessary, an up-dated statement is prepared) that we gleaned any information about Helen's rights under the 1981 Education Act. Had an honest statement of her special needs been drawn up (as, by law, it should have been) nine years previously we might have found it easier to ensure that her needs (for example for physiotherapy, the provision of which is, in this area, very poor) were addressed and met.

However, even though we were much better informed when, as Helen entered her teens, the time came for her special needs to be reviewed, it proved far from easy to get the authorities to approach their task with concern, honesty, thoroughness and speed. Indeed, such were their tardiness and disregard for their statutory obligations that we were forced to appeal to a tribunal to get an honest and full statement of Helen's needs and then some provision based on these. The experience was dispiriting, time-consuming and exhausting and although the tribunal found overwhelmingly in our favour against the Local Education Authority and Health Authority and, indeed, made strong recommendations as to how the authorities should improve their inadequate service, our feeling of satisfaction was diluted by our physical and emotional exhaustion.

Some years before this we had had another taste of how impossible it is to rely on the services on which you are dependent. Helen travels to and from the special unit she attends in an ambulance provided by Social Services. Although the present transport service functions well and is very reliable, this was not previously the case. Initially, and for several years, Helen travelled to and from the unit in a very old and battered taxi, the transport provided for her by the Local Education Authority. Because this vehicle frequently broke down, was unreliable and certainly looked unsound, we became increasingly concerned about its safety and roadworthiness. On several occasions Richard telephoned the Local Education Authority and he also wrote to ask what measures were taken to check on the safety of the vehicles used by their contractors for school transport. He was repeatedly fobbed off. One afternoon, while Helen was being driven home from the special unit, a wheel came off the taxi as it was driving along a main road. Helen, in her wheel-chair, was thrown sideways and left bruised, shaken and very distressed. Surely you are not being demanding if you expect that services provided (in this case for very vulnerable individuals) should be at the very least safe?

It is sometimes said that the test of a civilized society is the way in which it treats its elderly, disabled and sick. Sadly, through Helen's tragedy and Helen House, we have got to know many families whose difficulties and circumstances have heightened our awareness of how far from civilized (by this criterion) our society is. Our approach needs to be overhauled, our attitudes refined. Very often the needs of the disabled are overlooked in basic planning which inevitably makes disabled people feel at the least frustrated and more often marginalized or discounted. Disabled they may be, but citizens they yet remain, so that one wonders how the treatment meted out to them would be viewed in the light of the Citizen's Charter.

It would be naive to suppose that resources are unlimited. Many needs will inevitably remain unmet, particularly those in the life-enhancing, as opposed to life-sustaining, field. I have heard it argued that the failure to meet needs arises from people's re-classification of 'need', from the fact that people expect more and are being more demanding. It is probably true that people's expectations are greater; is this not inevitable as society progresses? Be that as it may, there are undoubtedly some problems which need to be addressed which do not stem simply from raised or unreal expectations.

The first is that major changes in provision under Care in the Community have been made with insufficient recognition of the resource implication of such changes. Care in the community is not cheap. This is perhaps forgotten (or glossed over) the more easily because neither of the two words 'care' and 'community' has immediate financial connotations.

Secondly, some of the professionals whose job it is to assess need and on whose assessment any subsequent provision or help for an ill, needy or disabled person will depend are reluctant to make a clear and unambiguous assessment of need. Their argument is that the resources are usually not available to provide for the need and that therefore nothing is achieved by stating the need. Quite apart from the fact that it is hard to see how they feel they can retain their professional credibility if they act in this way, this Alice-in-Wonderland approach ('I won't say it is there and then it isn't there') can have grave consequences for the ill and disabled. If those who have the expertise and knowledge and whose opinion carries weight, in short those who are perhaps more likely to be listened to at national level, choose not to highlight needs, there is little chance that adequate resources will ever be made available to meet the needs of the disabled and vulnerable.

A further sad consequence of professionals taking this attitude is that in doing so they make confrontation and conflict inevitable where there should be co-operation. How often I have been to meetings where suspicion and confrontation have completely stifled dialogue and openness. Parents of children with special needs, the sick, the disabled and the professionals in the 'caring professions' are surely united in their desire to obtain adequate resources and facilities. We all want the same thing. It is sad that some professionals seem to feel that it is 'rocking the boat' honestly to identify and state a need that cannot, in the existing climate, be met.

What is difficult for many disabled people, and also many families caring for an ill or handicapped child, is the way in which catering for the needs of these very vulnerable people is thought increasingly to be the role of charities, not the duty of society, through state provision. Voluntary-sector organizations, such as Age Concern, Mencap and the National Schizophrenia Fellowship and others have voiced their concern about this trend in connection with what they see as the under-funding of community care. They have expressed concern that what were formally government responsibilities are now being loaded onto charities. 'What we want is rights, not charity', is an understandable cry when you consider that many of the things increasingly often provided not by the state but by charities (and provision of which is therefore dependent upon the unpredictable charitable impulses and whims of individuals) are things that ill or disabled people desperately need simply to survive or live a reasonably pain-free or comfortable life. Moreover, if ill and disabled people have to depend on ad hoc fund-raising for provision of basic equipment and services the implications for their peace and privacy are serious. To encourage people to raise funds for him, the ill or disabled person often has to sacrifice his privacy and take on an (often unwelcome) public role.

On a more general note, if you have a very ill or disabled relative the choice between help and privacy is one that confronts you daily. Of course, it is more of a problem for some people than for others, because people value their privacy to very varying degrees. However, for some people the choice is a difficult one and the invasion of their privacy that being a carer brings with it is something they find hard to accept. Some people simply do not like holding open house to care assistants, nurses and social workers. Moreover, they find it upsetting to have to reveal all sorts of things about themselves and their circumstances so that their needs can be assessed. An added frustration is that their doing so does not necessarily result in their getting any help. Moreover, promises that they can check the information gathered about them (and their family) are not always honoured, as we have discovered from personal experience. What in these days of open access to information should be axiomatic, often, in practice, proves very difficult.

Reflections on Years of Caring

What is perhaps even harder to stomach is that much help for ill, handicapped or disabled individuals is now linked to popular mass entertainment. Quite apart from being patronizing, this approach has a very obvious danger attached to it. Entertainment is something you can take or leave as you choose, so, by tying in basic provision for the ill or disabled with mass entertainment, you remove that provision from the mainstream, you suggest that it is somehow 'optional', a peripheral, rather than a fundamental, concern. Very often, too, where help for the sick and disabled is linked to popular entertainment, the problems they face are trivialized and putting them across in such a way as to increase awareness, understanding and support comes a poor second to the promotion of the programme presenter's or the participating celebrities' 'good sport' or 'caring' image.

There is, too, evidence to suggest that charities like Children in Need and the Telethon Appeal, which were set up to enhance the basic provision for vulnerable children, children with special needs and the disabled are in fact not necessarily always adding to the funds available to help these groups but are increasingly replacing funds previously made available by local authorities or Health Authorities. As a governor of a special school I have seen examples of this. Because charities will sometimes provide, the official bodies whose duty it has traditionally been to make provision feel they do not always need to do so. The losers, ultimately, are those on the receiving (or non-receiving) end – those often least able to protect their interests.

At the start of National Integration Week in 1992 reference was made in a radio broadcast to 'the disabled and their supporters' – a strange remark, particularly in the context of integration! If the disabled and chronically sick are to be fully integrated into society they cannot be seen as objects of charity, a separate group that it is left to people to 'support' or not as they choose. We are all, if integration is to mean anything, their 'supporters'.

Of course I do not wish in any way to belittle the benevolence

207

and hard work of many people who work tirelessly to raise money for the helpless, disabled or vulnerable. I realize, too, that fundraising for a good cause generates a great deal of goodwill, creates friendships and, moreover, is something people enjoy and from which they derive enormous satisfaction. What I do believe (in common, I know, with many other families caring for a sick or disabled person) is that such fundraising should be for the provision of the 'icing on the cake' items, not for the basic cake itself.

If basic provision is left dependent upon people's charitable impulses then there is the obvious danger that only those individuals or initiatives that can be attractively or poignantly presented will get support. Linked to this is the way in which you can get people to support a children's hospice but will find it much harder to get people to think about the day-to-day problems of families caring at home over a long period of time for a very ill or disabled child. There is a parallel here in the world of medicine; heart surgery has more 'glamour' than, for example, rheumatism research; the obvious 'life and death flavour' of the former makes it seem much more important and worthy of support than the other, which is to do with a common, ongoing affliction. However, ironically, it is often the same children and families who attract great sympathy and 'tug at the heart strings' when focused on in the context of Helen House or another children's hospice, who battle with immensely draining but ongoing and rather unglamorous problems at home without attracting any great sympathy or support.

Put crudely, dying (or a dramatic illness or tragedy) attracts more sympathy than living on, albeit often increasingly helplessly and with premature death a certainty. Furthermore, death by its very finality perhaps defines people's roles and responses more clearly and is therefore, in that way at least, easier to cope with.

In Oscar Wilde's play *The Importance of Being Earnest* the formidable Lady Bracknell utters some very telling lines to her wayward nephew Algernon. Algernon has invented an invalid friend called Bunbury whose recurrent ill health he uses as an excuse when he does not want to attend some particularly tiresome social function. At one point in the first act Algernon tells his Aunt Augusta (Lady Bracknell) that he cannot come to her dinner party that evening because he has got to rush to Bunbury's bedside. His aunt's reply is swift:

'Well, I must say, Algernon, that I think it is high time that this Mr Bunbury made up his mind whether he was going to live or die. This shilly-shallying with the question is absurd. Nor do I in any way approve of the modern sympathy with invalids. I consider it morbid. Illness of any kind is hardly a thing to be encouraged in others. Health is the primary duty of life.'

Lady Bracknell is a person who likes things to be clearly defined. She likes things to be black or white. For her, things are either splendid or deplorable; there are no 'in-between' states. But the 'shilly-shallying' she so dislikes, the hovering between two absolutes, inevitably occurs with the long-term ill, those who do not make it clear to you where you stand or define your position by being conveniently clearly very alive or definitely dead. The long-term ill live in a twilight area and by the prolonged and often uncertain nature of their illness they force you, if you are going to remain in contact with them, to adapt your life and your attitudes to embrace this 'half-way state'. Their condition can be very embarrassing. It is, I would suggest, particularly embarrassing if they are children.

Most children who die after infancy die as a result of an accident. Their death is usually sudden and quick and therefore the shilly-shallying that so irritated Lady Bracknell is not usually a problem. Of course there is the awfulness, the unnaturalness of a child's death which is devastating to all involved. For a child to die before his parents is quite simply an affront against the natural order. But there is not, with a sudden death, this

209

twilight period where you have to work out your attitude to the invalid or the very sick person and sustain this over a period of time.

Many people are good in an emergency; fewer are good with a long-term tragedy or problem, though the difficulties and pain this problem causes those closely caught up in it may be every bit as acute as those caused by a sudden traumatic event. The ongoing support needed is what many people find it difficult to sustain. It is not simply that seeing someone in an acutely tragic situation is awkward because it makes you feel you 'ought' to be doing something to help when perhaps you do not actually want to; to suggest that this is the most common feeling is to fail to credit people with the compassion and fellow feeling many of them undoubtedly have.

I think that for most people the idea that a fellow human being could be suffering and distressed over a very long period of time quite simply does not bear thinking about. That we have a deep-seated psychological need to extend the soothing 'There there, better now', of our childhood into situations we find ourselves in in adulthood is clear; tell-tale signs of this creep out all the time in what we say, whether privately or more publicly. Soon after we brought Helen home from hospital, a friend who was very upset at what had happened to Helen, and who felt for us deeply, told me one day that I should feel free to come and collapse on her from time to time if I felt the need. She then added, 'I don't know how long I'll be able to take it for, though. Well, I don't know what any of us will feel able to do if Helen is still in the same state in a couple of years' time.' Our pain and problems would then simply not bear thinking about.

Recently a news report a week after an elderly man and his daughter had been brutally murdered and their bodies dismembered, focused on an appeal to the public to help catch the killer by the fiancé of the murdered young woman. The report stated: 'A week after the murders, Mr X has still not come to terms with the tragedy.' Only a great need to think the murdered woman's fiancé was not suffering acutely, to feel he was 'better now', could make us find the word 'still' appropriate in that sentence.

Because people find a long-drawn-out tragedy difficult, if that is what engulfs your life you feel very isolated. You do not get even the understanding a bereaved person gets (and I know very well that that understanding, sympathy and support is often fleeting) because you are not, technically, bereaved. However, any parent of a very sick or disabled child has suffered a loss – the loss of the happy, well child of their dreams, the child that in this high-tech age most people have come to see as their right. In our case we have lost the Helen we once knew, and also day by day we know and feel the loss of the Helen our beloved eldest daughter once seemed destined to become. I remember vividly the day Helen's friends from her 'well days' and nursery music class started infant school. That day I felt acutely the loss of a bright-eyed, eager little girl with highly-polished shoes, proudly clasping a lunch box and a pencil case. We have felt other, similar losses over the years more times than I could count.

The words 'isolated' and 'isolation' crop up again and again when parents of very ill or disabled children describe their feelings. Although there is growing awareness nowadays of the needs and problems of carers, these carers are typically looking after elderly parents, partners or relatives. Recent surveys indicate that sixty-one per cent of those cared for at home are in the sixty-five to eighty-five age group while only three per cent are in the under-sixteen age group. The plight of parents caring for a very ill child does not really impinge on public awareness and, where it does, it often, as I said earlier, causes embarrassment. Children, after all, are supposed to be irrepressibly lively and active; they are, as we are always being told, our future.

If you have problems caring for, organizing provision or making arrangements for, your frail, elderly mother you will probably find a lot of people are sympathetic and identify with your difficulties, either because they are, or have been, in the same situation themselves or because they realize they might be in the future. Read house sale advertisements and you will soon find mention of a 'granny flat' or a 'granny annexe'. These words have entered the language because they describe a common need. Caring for a helpless or frail child is, by contrast, not a situation many people have, or will have, experience of. Moreover, if you are in this situation you are a 'carer' often at a stage in your life when, because of their combined experience and energy, most people expect to live life most fully, not to be severely restricted. Many things you might normally expect to be taking on fairly easily (and which your friends and contemporaries perhaps are) are beyond you.

One of the things we find hardest about our life with Helen is the way we have to make elaborate plans and arrangements to make even quite ordinary outings and excursions possible. I have quite a strong impulsive streak and I find not being free to act spontaneously very irksome. Planned spontaneity is somehow not quite the same! Also, our outings (if they are without Helen) come to depend very much on the free time, availability and goodwill of the few people who are able and willing to care for Helen in our absence. Moreover, we have to plan a very long time ahead if we want to go away for a weekend on our own or take a holiday with only Catherine and Isobel. Since there is so much uncertainty surrounding Helen, both day to day (on some days she is much less well than on others; some days she is very disturbed and has more frequent seizures) and on a longer time-scale (we do not know how long she will live) to be so certain of one's own plans is very difficult and indeed making plans seems somehow inappropriate or 'tempting fate'.

Exhaustion is a great problem for us, particularly since we simply do not have the time (or backup support) to go under! Caring for Helen day in, day out is extremely tiring and even when she is at her most serene and relaxed her basic needs (dressing, feeding, changing, washing, medication, gentle exercising of limbs, changing of position) obviously still need to be attended to. We do all these tasks very willingly and indeed doing them lovingly brings us comfort, for one of the most painful things about Helen's condition is the way it greatly limits our opportunities for doing things or giving her things which will bring her real joy or pleasure. Yet, however positively we approach the tasks we undertake for Helen and however willingly we undertake them, they are nonetheless draining. They are all the more so because of the heavy undertow of grief that is always there, sapping our energy. We are most strongly aware of the presence of this undertow when we stop (usually briefly, perhaps for a short break) doing all the things we do for Helen, and have time to reflect. It is often in these periods of respite that grief overwhelms us. Holidays with Helen's two sisters are precious but also times when the awfulness of what has happened to Helen comes home to us. On holiday we no longer have the execution of oft-recurring tasks to keep us busy and take our minds off what has happened to Helen, and it is often when we are on holiday that our sense of bereavement is most acute. On holiday, too, we are struck by how long a day is when the hours are not regularly eroded by the demands of our role as 'carers'. When on holiday we often wonder, too, whether we will ever have the energy to resume our regular lifestyle when the holiday is over.

Of course, there are moments when we are not on holiday when we feel utterly bereft, when we suddenly feel over-whelmed by sorrow, and these moments can occur at any time, often completely unexpectedly and for no obvious reason. There is little logic or predictability in grieving. Penelope Lively sums this up beautifully in her novel *Perfect Happiness*:

> Grief like illness is unstable; it ebbs and flows in tides, it steals away to a distance and then comes roaring back, it torments by deception. It plays games with time and with reality.

She also touches on the loneliness of those who grieve when she says: 'Unhappiness isolates; grief is not contagious.'

Paradoxical as this may sound, unpredictability is something you have to be prepared for when you are looking after a child who is very ill or disabled. You cannot count on unbroken nights or seizure-free days; your child may, for no apparent reason, suddenly have a bad day or be very disturbed or even very ill. Such spells may pass as quickly as they came. The strain of such ups and downs is hard to describe, as is the physical and emotional exhaustion you feel when your child has come close to death and then suddenly picked up. Holding yourself in readiness at one and the same time for a death which may well not occur and for carrying on as before with the same energy and determination, requires immense reserves of strength.

When you are facing what sometimes seem like insurmountable problems day after day and sometimes feel quite crushed by them, you sometimes long for a little help from those around you. Unless you ask, though, (and to keep asking is difficult) all but the very sensitive will probably not offer, not because they are unkind, thoughtless or uncaring, but because in their eyes the length of time you have lived with your problem somehow dilutes its acuteness. You *have* coped, therefore obviously you *can* cope. I think people in situations like ours are on a losing wicket here; if they cope well or simply adequately it is assumed that the coping is effortless and they do not need help. We emerge from our house looking calm, with Helen in her wheelchair looking (we hope) lovely. How can people (except the really imaginative) know what lies behind this picture? I am sure there must be many parents in situations like ours who emerge, like Eleanor Rigby, 'wearing a face that they keep in a jar by the door'. I suspect, though, that if they came out looking distraught, distressed and in no way in control, this would put people off and be more likely to isolate them than to generate support.

Sometimes people's praise of how you manage, though it

214

can be cheering in one sense, is unhelpful in another in that it makes you feel you cannot unsettle them by suggesting that you are not really managing and could do with some help. Their praise is paralysing; you feel you most go on doing well if only for their sake. Alison, the mother of a disabled child, Molly, in Margaret Drabble's *The Ice Age* knows the feeling well:

> A wonderful woman and a wonderful mother. Yes. Alison stared at the two airmail letters. People were always describing her as a wonderful woman and a wonderful mother. Why? Because she let Molly come home for the holidays, instead of dumping her all the year round, as so many did? Or in the hope that, if so described, she would continue so to behave?

Richard and I both have jobs we enjoy and other interests and commitments outside the home which we would not wish to give up. Since he took up his present post as The Government Chemist, Richard has increasingly often been away from home and therefore unable to help as much as he would wish with Helen's day-to-day care. Furthermore, of course, we have two daughters in addition to Helen. Keeping a balance between our needs, Helen's needs and her sisters' needs is not easy and nor is finding time and energy for all the things we want to do and leading a normal life. Of course, we must not forget that for Catherine and Isobel normal life is life with Helen as she now is; they have never known anything different. This in itself can bring problems, perhaps the greatest of these being how we address the subject of Helen's uncertain life span. I realized when Catherine and Isobel were still quite small that Helen was so naturally incorporated in our family, so much part of us, that her sisters in a sense forgot that she was in any way ill or frail and took it for granted that she would always be with us. I did not wish to stifle the (to us very cheering) naturalness of their approach to Helen nor

215

to introduce wariness or anxiety where none (happily) seemed to exist. Equally, though Helen's death would undoubtedly be a shock for all of us whenever it occurred, I did not want it to happen without the *possibility* of it happening unexpectedly having been introduced to Catherine and Isobel. I would not wish them to feel that we had been secretive or had misled them about Helen's condition; trust between parents and children is always important but in situations which are made uncertain or precarious by circumstances beyond our control and where insecurity can easily creep in, this trust is even more important.

Rather than seeking to 'create' opportunities to introduce the idea that Helen might die before the rest of us, I try to use those which arise naturally. For example, some years ago when Catherine and Isobel were still quite small we were talking about a friend's wedding. Catherine said that if/when she got married Isobel and Helen would be her bridesmaids. Seeing Helen's inability to walk as the only possible problem, she said, 'Helen could wear a lovely dress and you could push her in her wheelchair.' I agreed that it was a lovely idea 'if Helen is still alive then'.

The word 'partnership' is currently a buzz word in the field of education and health care. We hear much about 'partnership with parents' and professionals can even be heard to say that 'parents are the experts'. From this it should surely follow that the professionals and the providers listen to parents. Sadly, however, the statement 'parents are the experts' is often used as an excuse, a justification for leaving parents to do everything for themselves, even those things professionals receive training to master. Again, partnership suggests some measure of equality, yet often, even in non-professional fields, the views of parents are not accorded anything approaching the weight given to those of professionals. Just as, in the old saying, 'gentlemen perspire and ladies merely glow', professionals 'know', parents merely 'have perceptions'!

Related to this is the assumption that because of your

problem or tragedy you are firmly fixed in all ways in a subordinate position, you are passive, the person things are done to (or not done to!), the hapless victim of current theories and practices. (In the professional field this hardly accords with the notion of partnership; on the personal/friendship level it sits ill with notions of true friendship, which involve seeing friendship as rooted in equality.) The language so often used, even where there is genuine concern, reveals this to be the case. 'We must give parents permission to grieve'; only those who are in a superior position, or a position of authority over you, can 'give you permission'! 'Let' is the appropriate word here: 'We must let parents grieve', i.e. simply do nothing to stand in the way of what they may need or want to do.

Letting people in very unhappy or difficult circumstances do what is most helpful to them is very important. To be prescriptive about what they should or should not want to do is unhelpful. In this connection the certainty and unquestioning confidence of some professionals that they know exactly what the feelings of, for example, the bereaved or the parents of very ill children are, and that they know what is 'right' or 'therapeutic' for them is quite breathtaking at times. Individuals are so different and react in such different ways that although you may perhaps be able to say that often (even usually) parents experience certain feelings, you cannot say this is how *all* parents feel. If you do say this, far from giving the help you probably wish to give, you may greatly increase the isolation and unhappiness of those who do not in fact feel as you assume they do.

Some people in very unhappy situations find it helpful to pour out their feelings; others do not. It is undoubtedly a good thing that nowadays there is much more openness, much more awareness of feelings, much more understanding of some people's need to talk about their emotions and fears. However, in this climate it is important to remember the needs of those who do not find it helpful to talk about their innermost feelings. 'Helping them to express these' is not necessarily the answer;

your zeal to help them 'let it all hang out' may in fact leave them feeling utterly wretched at what they have been forced to reveal, or to claim they feel, in order to conform to your stereotype.

On a personal note, people have sometimes asked me if I am 'angry with God' because of what has happened to Helen. I find this completely meaningless. I feel many things in relation to what has happened to Helen – among them immense sadness, pity, wistfulness – but not, and never, anger. But I (and others like me) cannot win here. If we say we do not feel anger we are told we are suppressing it. Or, if we say we feel anger about some things – injustice, the inadequacies of provision for the vulnerable, frail and helpless – then we hear that this, of course, is the anger we feel about the tragedy in our life, that is seeking an outlet somewhere else!

To the other question I am sometimes asked in relation to the supposed anger I must feel about what has happened to Helen, whether I do not often rant and rave and ask, 'Why me? Why should such a tragedy befall *my* daughter?' I can only say that I have never spontaneously asked myself this question but when it is put to me by others I can only say, 'Why *not* me?'

The feeling of isolation families caring for a very ill child experience is often intensified by the language the professionals use and by the jargon they seem so fond of. Much of this 'cushioning' language, which shuns concrete facts and simple statements is undoubtedly funny. (We do not 'do things for ourselves' – we 'adopt a self-help mentality'; we do not 'cope' – we 'utilize our coping mechanisms'; we are never in or at a specific place, 'at home', 'at school' – we are 'in a home situation', 'in a school situation'.) The trouble with this 'padded language' beloved of those organizing the 'caring services' is that by its very padded nature it insulates those who use it against what it is supposed to describe, distances them and soon prohibits action. Its imprecision blurs the sharp focus that the needs of the vulnerable need to be in.

Many families who visit Helen House have stories to tell

about difficulties they have had communicating with the 'caring professions' and getting their ideas and needs across. Many, too, describe difficulties with the medical profession and how difficult they find it to talk to doctors who 'shut them out' by using language of an inappropriately and starkly specialist variety even in casual conversation. The language of the text book spills over into even social exchanges. One parent suggested one day that perhaps doctors (like many others) find directness threatening because it means they need to get involved. It is hardly surprising that a mother grieving the death of her young son says she feels she simply cannot talk to her doctor or ask him for help since the day when her breaking down in tears in his surgery provoked the measured statement, 'Premature mortality is indeed traumatic.'

As I have said before, your interests and tastes do not usually change because you have been overtaken by tragedy or have a great problem to contend with. You may have considerably less time to pursue your interests and indulge your tastes, but these remain the same and continue to a great extent to determine your conductor and your life-style. However, it does seem that there are those who would link everything that you or your family do or say to the (admittedly enormous) problem or tragedy in your life and interpret it accordingly.

This was in part the reason that Richard and I felt uneasy about a research project led by a consultant paediatrician which was initiated when Helen House had been open for three years. The initial stated objectives of the research study were startlingly ambitious: To assess 'the impact of chronic, life-threatening illness on the family' and the role of Helen House 'in mitigating this impact as compared with NHS care'. Other objectives were to identify the major stresses experienced by the staff at Helen House and to review facilities available for respite care of children in England and Wales. The study was to be set up like a clinical trial of a drug with twenty-five children and their families who used Helen House being matched with a similar group not using the hospice. An assessment was to be made of 'the families' psycho-social functioning, including general health, marital adjustment, coping and sibling involvement'.

The leader of the study saw it as being sufficiently important that he wrote to *The Times* (25th March 1986) to 'urge restraint on those who are considering establishing a local children's hospice'. He concluded: 'A new service is no different from a new drug; we should not unleash it wholesale on the community at large until we have defined by careful research the therapeutic advantages, side effects and indications for the innovation.' In his letter he argued that Helen House had been a result of 'guesswork' and the further development of children's hospices was 'problematical'.

While Richard and I felt that an assessment of need and a review of available facilities was clearly desirable, we had serious misgivings about whether the main objectives of the study could be met using the methodology proposed. We felt that conclusions based on a statistical analysis of inevitably different families in such a small sample would not be sound. We had doubts about the attempts to *quantify*, for example, sibling involvement and then construct a causal link with just one common factor, the severe illness of a brother or sister. Of course, the 'psycho-social functioning' of a family (even if one accepts, which we do not, that this is a quantifiable, rather than descriptive, phenomenon) is likely to be greatly influenced by the serious illness of a child, but there are other factors, such as simply a commonly occurring fact that the parents are not getting on with each other or that a child has changed schools or that the family has moved, that can also have a significant effect! As Tolstoy puts it: 'All happy families are alike, but each unhappy family is unhappy in its own way.'

However, it was the very public plea that the foundation of further children's hospices should be halted until the results of this (in our view, rather unsoundly-based) research project were available that we felt went beyond the remit of Helen House. In his letter to *The Times* the project leader had signed as 'Chairman, Helen House Research Steering Committee'. We felt it was unprofessional for a supposedly objective study of hospice care to be associated with Helen House in this way. The study of supermarkets by one major retailer would not necessarily be regarded as objective and independent! Helen House is in fact a model of hospice care; but suppose it were not? Would the Helen House study of children's hospice care then be any more credible than the Lowood study of children's educational establishments?

Although our inclination had always been not to correct what was published in the press on Helen House, judging our privacy to be more important than putting the record straight, we felt on this occasion, and after much soul-searching, that we had to reply to the letter. In our response, which was published in *The Times*, we supported the sensible points about the need to consider carefully the demand for children's hospices and their geographical distribution but we questioned the 'unfortunate analogies between the provision of respite care in hospices and drug therapy'. We recorded that the starting point for Helen House was not a medical one and that Helen House had stemmed from the desire to provide respite care and friendship to families like ours in home-like surroundings. Though there were uncertainties surrounding its birth, there was never any 'guesswork' involved in what it should be like. We concluded: '[The] use of terminology such as "undesirable side effects" is as inappropriate in this context as has been some of the over-sentimental coverage given to Helen House in the popular press. In his anxiety to curb a possible outbreak of hospice founding, induced perhaps by such publicity, [your correspondent] misses the opportunity to point out that hospice care is only one aspect of the support which the community could offer.'

Friendly and open discussions with those involved in the research study did not dispel our serious reservations about the scope and structure of the exercise. However, it was later accepted that the warnings given in the letter to *The Times* over children's hospice care were made largely in ignorance of the patchiness and dearth of other support services for children with life-threatening illnesses and their families.

No one could take issue with the often obvious but nonetheless valid conclusions of those involved in the research study, which have now been published. Those involved in the project approached their task with great sensitivity and gained considerable insight into the work of Helen House and the feelings of the staff who work there. It is good (though startling that they need to be) that doctors and other readers of medical literature should be reminded that 'the impact of chronic life-threatening illness on the families [studied] was substantial' and that, when the diagnosis of a life-threatening illness was being imparted to them, parents 'disliked evasive or unsympathetic brief interviews'. The authors' call for better information on the range and availability of current services and material provision will strike a chord with many parents. A positive outcome has been the collection of such a data base by ACT (Action for the Care of families whose children have life-threatening and Terminal Conditions).

However, we have always felt that a quantitative measure of the 'efficacy' of Helen House compared with 'regular health service provision' has little meaning, not least because the 'regular health service provision' is so variable that it can hardly be defined. It was never the intention of Helen House to *duplicate* existing home care facilities (or for that matter mimic paediatric wards); rather, Helen House is a modest venture to complement existing provision and to provide respite care to parents and their children.

Our misgivings about this type of socio-medical research are more general. Results arising from the use of indices, scales and questionnaires often need to be interpreted with considerable caution, particularly when you are dealing with small samples. It is frightening how conclusions are sometimes stated with such authority when they are based on such fragile foundations. Taken to extremes (and I am not referring here to research on hospice care) the unquestioning application of such research has overridden common sense with disastrous consequences, as graphically recorded in the Butler-Sloss enquiry into child abuse in Cleveland.

In an age when every home computer in the country is capable of spewing out pages of figures, and when the phrase 'research has shown that' is used to add gravitas to even the most banal observations, we realize that it is swimming against the tide to suggest that clear thinking, consistent use of language and, when statistics are gathered, consideration of uncertainty and error, should be essential tools of research in this field. However, it is surprising to us that reputable medical journals do not insist on an elementary consideration of measurement uncertainty as an essential element of studies which draw conclusions from statistical data. Rather, one can get the impression that a mass of undigested figures is a pre-requisite to publication!

When we first brought Helen home from hospital six months after her major operation the neurosurgeon who had operated on her said he felt it was unlikely that she would live for more than a few years. He felt that it was quite possible that she would succumb to an infection of some sort. He has said to us on several occasions since then that the fact that Helen has lived so long is a great tribute to us and the way we care for her. While it helps us to think that an objective observer feels we look after Helen well – for we often feel we do not do nearly enough for her – at the same time we find it painful to think that Helen owes her extended life span to us. Her present life is such a twilight existence that we cannot help asking ourselves what we are giving our beloved Helen. Yet, of course, we could never slacken in our efforts to care for her as well as it is in our power to do; such is our love for her that we could never give her anything less than the best we are able to offer.

It is natural when people are upset or unhappy to try to cheer them up and in doing so people often resort to well-worn phrases and clichés. One such is 'Every cloud has a silver lining'. Obviously it is sensible to try to focus on the positive in life and this is certainly my inclination generally. However, the use of the 'silver lining' saying is really only appropriate where the cloud is a minor setback or a relatively insignificant inconvenience; its use in the context of serious tragedy or illness is bound to cause pain. In our case, the saying could be said to have a very obvious significance; something very wonderful and of immense benefit to others has resulted from Helen's tragedy. Helen's and our personal cloud has a silver lining that shines well beyond our small circle. However, despite the exceptional quality of the silver lining, it does not in any way dispel the cloud. The huge cloud remains.

A cliché which has a lot of relevance for us is the old saying 'You have to laugh or you'd cry'. Over the years that we have cared for Helen at home the jargon, bureaucratic zeal, unquestioning application of rules across the board, the inflexible attitudes, the ever-increasing numbers of co-ordinators and liaison persons and the general lack of common sense that pervades the whole process of providing care and support to the frail, elderly and sick – these have placed us at times in quite ridiculous and even funny situations. However, though the text may at times be richly comic, the sub-text remains deeply sad.

A few months ago we took Helen to Cornwall with her sisters and back to the beautiful beach where she had splashed so happily at the age of eight months. It was a poignant pilgrimage, all the more so since it was to Cornwall that we had been about to take Helen for a holiday the day she was so suddenly taken ill in 1978. While I was sitting with Helen one day in beautiful Trelissick Gardens, watching Catherine and Isobel climb a huge tree, I got into conversation with two women sitting on the garden seat beside me. In the course of our conversation they asked me if Catherine and Isobel 'were understanding'. I was not sure exactly what they meant and I have pondered on the question often since. At a basic level

Catherine and Isobel understand (that is to say know the facts about) what happened to Helen. On the other hand they no more understand the why of what has befallen their sister than we do. If by 'understanding' the two women meant (as I think they probably did) that Catherine and Isobel do not blame Helen for the restrictions she imposes on our life, then I think I can say that they do not see her in those terms, much to their credit. Their love of Helen far outweighs (as far as I can tell, anyway) any irritation, embarrassment or (dare I say it!) anger they might feel. If Helen is noisy, Catherine can feel as cross as she would feel if she was disturbed by Isobel. I find this reassuring.

What is certain is that Helen is loved beyond measure. We never feel we do enough for her and will always try to do more. Life is often hard and we sometimes feel utterly exhausted, lonely and at times overwhelmed by sadness. Yet, (to borrow a phrase from Jacqueline du Pré, tapes of whose cello playing we often put on for Helen) I feel that I really am a very lucky person. I do not feel this *because* of what has happened to Helen; I cannot go along with the idea that I am privileged to have suffered as I have because I am ennobled by suffering, I am somehow a better person for it. I feel I am lucky because the past fourteen years have not robbed me of my enthusiasm; I still feel a great zest for life. Richard and I are very close, our daughters bring us immense joy, we have full and rewarding lives and many good friends. I am a lucky person.

Of course, I cannot help feeling wistful from time to time and thinking 'If only . . .' but stronger than this is always 'Yes, in spite of all'.

Conclusion

Much has changed in the long years since Helen first became ill. Many of the changes have been positive and perhaps indicate a welcome return to basic human values. In the field of medicine there are signs of a more holistic approach in the treatment of the sick and injured. There is a growing awareness of the connection between physical and emotional well-being, of the fact that the noun 'patient' is descriptive only of an ill or injured individual's role or position *vis-à-vis* a doctor or nurse and is not a general substitute for 'human being'. Thus it seems to be more widely recognized now that concern and care for the person, the human being, can influence greatly the success of the medical treatment offered to 'the patient'.

Things which basic common sense and instinct would tell you are helpful and good are now coming into mainstream medical care. An interesting example of this is something which was adopted quite naturally at Helen House from the start, though without being spelt out or described – the idea of the 'named person'. Increasingly in hospitals one member of staff, known to the patient by name, assumes responsibility for all aspects of that patient's care and thus has the chance to get to know the patient and, it is hoped, meet his needs more effectively and sensitively.

Not long ago the National Association for the Welfare of Children in Hospital was renamed; it is now called Action for Sick Children. This marks a recognition of the role played by parents and families in the care of sick children, of the fact that serious illness is not encountered, and indeed treated or coped with, only within the confines of hospitals. The chairman of the Oxfordshire branch of ASC said in a news interview in November 1991 that the new name marked changes in the care offered to children. 'Advances in modern medicine and

226

treatment mean that in the nineties children are spending less time as in-patients in hospital. This means that parents are having to play a greater role in the nursing of their sick children.' As a result, ASC aims to forge closer links with hospital staff, community health workers and parents 'to ensure that families are properly informed and supported through this difficult time'.

There have been changes, too, in society more generally. There is certainly a greater awareness now of the problems confronting those caring at home for the frail, elderly, sick or disabled. Although many of these 'carers' unfortunately still get no chance to take a break from their exhausting task, respite care, which fifteen years ago was hardly talked about, is now recognized as an integral part of the provision which, properly, should be available to those 'caring in the community'. Funding and provision, sadly, do not always follow awareness but recognizing a problem is the first step towards addressing it and solving it and we must hope that provision will not lag too far behind awareness.

In the field of care of those with life-threatening illness and of the terminally ill, adult hospices are now relatively commonplace and certainly no longer arouse the controversy they did in their pioneering days. When Helen House opened in 1982 there were no other children's hospices in the world; there are now five children's hospices in operation in England and seventeen planned. The number of families using them shows that there is a great need for respite care at all stages of life-threatening illness. Those who doubted that there was a significant need for children's hospices on the lines of Helen House misread the signs.

The opening of Helen House generated discussion in professional circles on the relative merits of care and support in their own homes for children with life-limiting illness and their families, and care and support in a hospice. We have always felt that setting the two types of support against each other, of adopting an either/or approach, was misguided.

A House Called Helen

There is ample room, indeed an overwhelming need, for both types of support, to meet not only the different needs of different families but also the different needs of the same families at different times.

Related to this is the philosophy versus facility argument. While it is undoubtedly true that the philosophy of care and support for the very ill needs to be broadened, it should never be supposed that because you have a philosophy you do not need a facility. The danger of this neat alliterative juxtaposition of philosophy and facility is that if the idea behind it were to be embraced literally, it could leave those in need of practical help deprived of such assistance, drowning in a sea of abstract terminology.

With attitudes changing and the hope therefore that there might be real improvements in provision and in the organization of services, we are aware that, in the field of care of children with life-threatening illness at least, Helen House is often looked to as a model. Indeed Helen House has been described as a model of hospice care and a centre of excellence. This is gratifying but carries risks. The very success of Helen House can lead people to imagine it is something more complicated than it is; nowadays we seem unable to link success with simplicity. Yet Helen House is a modest venture. It is not *the* answer; it is just *one* of the ways in which children with life-threatening illness and their families can be helped.

Helen House is now so well established and fulfils such an important function that it is hard to believe that there was ever a time when it did not exist. Yet the hospice is still comparatively young. Most of the people who were involved in its planning and who remember the thinking behind the important decisions relating to its size and function are still around and on hand to provide background information and to talk about the philosophy underlying the hospice. However, as time goes on this, inevitably, will not be the case. Moreover, there are bound to be changes in the staff and there will come a time when none of the original team is still working at Helen

House. There will be new people in the key positions of Head Nurse and Administrator.

To ensure that the original guiding philosophy is preserved and that the aims and beliefs are handed down clearly to those who in the future will be in charge of running the hospice, it was felt as the tenth anniversary approached that it would be a good idea to set up a small group of people called the Guardians of Helen House, whose role would be a guiding and overseeing one. The emphasis at Helen House has always been on human values and on informality. By calling the group 'Guardians', we wished to preserve the family analogy and to assume *vis-à-vis* Helen House the role the guardian of a child assumes in relation to that child.

The Statement of the Purpose and Responsibilities of the Guardians of Helen House runs as follows:

> The Guardians exist to offer advice to the Mother Superior with the aim of ensuring the continuing success of Helen House and the greatest well-being and happiness possible for the children, parents, relatives and bereaved who come to it, and the staff who work there. The Guardians provide a forum for discussing matters of policy which could have implications for the future of Helen House. They have a particular responsibility to assist the Mother Superior and staff of Helen House to sustain the underlying philosophy which has been expressed in the leaflets, regular newsletters and in the day-to-day running of Helen House over the last nine years. The Guardians are also available to offer advice to the Mother Superior over the appointment of the Head Nurse, the Administrator and the Medical Director. These three will be Guardians while they hold office at Helen House.

The Guardians have met about twice a year since the inaugural meeting in September 1991. We are a small group that includes those originally involved in the foundation of Helen House and others with a close interest in its operation. These include a parent and a representative of the Helen House team chosen by the team themselves.

Our first major task was the appointment of a successor to Edith Anthem as Head Nurse. Following external advertisements a short list of candidates was drawn up and interviews took place in November 1992. Everyone involved with Helen House was delighted when the one internal candidate for the post was selected. Mary Thompson took up her post as Head Nurse in April 1993.

People often talk to us of the pride we must feel at the great success of Helen House. As the tenth birthday of the hospice approached we certainly felt very moved at what had been achieved. For the service of thanksgiving to mark the occasion, Christ Church Cathedral in Oxford was full to capacity as the many families from all over the country who have used Helen House since it opened and the staff who have worked there came together and gave thanks. It was then, when we were surrounded by the 'Helen House families' that we felt proud at the success of Helen House, for by its success we do not mean simply its public acclaim but rather the fact that it has been able to help so many and such different families. This it has been able to do because of the simplicity of its approach and because its roots are firmly established in the fruitful terrain of love, humanity and common sense. We hope that in the years to come Helen House will remain thus rooted.

We do not know how long our beloved Helen will live. What we do know is that her influence will extend 'far beyond her years'.

9

Into the New Millennium

When I wrote the preceding chapters in 1993, the obvious need and lack of provision that Helen House had sought to address had already led others to set up children's hospices, broadly on the Helen House model. Martin House (Yorkshire) opened in 1987, Acorns (Birmingham) in 1988, the first two of East Anglia's children's hospices (Cambridge and Norfolk) in 1989 and 1991 respectively, and Francis House (Manchester) in 1991. What was not predicted, perhaps, was the increasing speed with which children's hospices would come into being during the final decade of the twentieth century, nor indeed the fact that, by their very numbers (not by their individual size), they would stimulate an appraisal of the whole area of care for children with life-limiting illnesses.

There are now twenty-two children's hospices in operation in the UK, with a further thirteen at the project stage. In addition there are two organizations (one in Hertfordshire, one in Surrey) which offer an exclusively home hospice service. All the hospices are small; none has more than eleven beds and the three units developed under the umbrella of an existing adult hospice are considerably smaller (two have four beds, one has two beds). Thus, all can be said to embrace the belief fundamental to Helen House, namely that small scale fosters flexibility, sensitivity and dignity.

Although the exact words chosen by individual hospices to describe their objectives vary – each hospice retains its own individuality and in no way does communality of purpose mean that children's hospices constitute a 'chain' – the philosophy which sustains them all remains essentially the same philosophy as that on which Helen House was founded.

231

Unifying the approach and establishing networks

In 1995 a group of representatives from six established children's hospices, aware of the increasing momentum towards the creation of children's hospices and the growing interest in this area of paediatric care, sought to set out this philosophy in a document entitled *Guidelines for Good Practice in a Children's Hospice*. Having begun by stating that the aim of a children's hospice was 'to offer holistic care for a child with a life-limiting condition and his or her family', the authors of the guidelines then proceed to make, and expand upon, a series of statements which they suggest clarify the core values central to the role and purpose of a children's hospice.

In their unexpanded form these are:

- The services offered by a children's hospice will be available to children and adolescents with a life-limiting condition and their families. No direct charge will be made to families.
- A children's hospice will provide a safe home-from-home environment.
- The care offered will aim to meet the social, cultural, spiritual, physical and emotional needs of the child and family.
- The care given will be guided by the wishes of the individual child and family, whether in the hospice or at home.
- Appropriate support will be made available to meet the needs of the family members and those closely involved with the child and his or her family.
- Symptom control will aim to promote comfort and enhance quality of life.
- Care will be continued during the terminal phase of the child's life and following death.
- Bereavement care will be available to the family.
- A high quality service will be maintained.

232

In their conclusions the authors recommend that these guidelines be used 'to influence the development of services aimed at the care of a child with a life-limiting illness and his or her family'. Thus, open expression was given for the first time to the importance of an approach to, and a style of, care, developed and fostered within the existing children's hospices, being extended into, and permeating, the full range of service provision for children with life-limiting illnesses.

It was from the deliberations of this small group of representatives (originally the Head Nurses/Heads of Care who had begun to meet together to share ideas and experience) that the Association of Children's Hospices was born. The Association was established as a registered charity in 1998 'for the benefit of the public to promote the interests of the children's hospice movement and, in particular, to develop public awareness and support of children's hospices and paediatric palliative care'.

The Association provides a very useful forum for discussion and debate. Representatives from member organizations meet regularly to share good practice, review their work, debate issues of current concern and consider how best to increase understanding (and thus uptake) of their services. Importantly, they can collectively, speaking with the authority of knowledge gained from experience in the field, act as an advisory, or cautionary, service for those seeking to establish hospice services for children.

One of the points that the Association has sought to put across most forcefully since its inception is that children's hospices are not simply mini adult hospices, that the ethos of the one is very different from that of the other, not least because of the (usually) considerably greater longevity of the ill children who use its services as compared with that of the patients in an adult hospice. (I discuss the differences between adult and children's hospices later in this chapter.) For this reason, the Association argues, children's hospices should be distinct and apart from adult ones, in separate and specially

designed accommodation. The Association is currently review-
ing its objectives and considering whether it should remain as
an essentially advisory body and forum for discussion, whether
it should promote itself more explicitly as the recognized
voice of children's hospices or whether it should take on a
more 'political' role, seeking to shape policy at the national
level.

The UK is widely recognized as the leader in the field where
children's hospices are concerned. In the UK alone there are
more free-standing hospices than exist in the whole of the rest
of the world. This is not to say that children's hospice care, by
which is meant a concept of holistic care that is not restricted
to any one setting, is not very much on the agenda worldwide. The number of hospice care programmes attached to
hospitals or paediatric units, or set up within the community,
is growing rapidly. Children's Hospice International, founded
in 1983 in Alexandria, Virginia, USA with the twin aims of
providing help and support to children with life-threatening
conditions and their families, and education, training and technical assistance to healthcare professionals, provides information on a wide range of such programmes. The strength of
children's hospice care, wherever it is delivered, lies in its
essentially 'co-operative' nature; it brings together a wide
range of individuals – doctors, nurses, teachers, therapists,
clergy, social workers, administrators and volunteers – who,
as a team, provide the care and support needed by children
facing premature death and their families.

There are now children's hospices in a number of other
countries, among them Australia, Canada, Germany and the
United States. What is exciting is to see the links that already
exist, forged both for professional reasons and through a
feeling of common purpose and friendship, between hospices
in different countries. Exchange of information, sharing of
good practice and mutual encouragement and support across
national boundaries can only benefit the development of
children's hospice care.

Canuck Place, which opened in Vancouver, British Columbia, Canada in November 1994 had strong links with Helen House in its planning stage; one of the prime movers in its foundation spent a number of months working in Helen House and used the experience and knowledge she gathered to inform the planning and development stage of the first Canadian children's hospice. Canuck Place has just become an Associate Member of the Association of Children's Hospices, thus strengthening links between paediatric palliative care in Canada and the UK.

Balthasar, the first continental European children's hospice, located in the small town of Olpe in the heart of the Sauerland in Germany, opened its doors in autumn 1998. The group of parents who originally came together ten years ago to discuss setting up a hospice in Germany heard of Helen House through the Mucopolysaccharidosis (MPS) Society. They established links through visits and subsequent communication. The young daughter of one couple came to Helen House for respite care and her parents thus had the opportunity to become familiar with the way the hospice operated. The philosophy and ethos at Balthasar is very similar to that of Helen House and the friendship between the two hospices is sustained by on-going contact between the staff of the two establishments.

One very happy example of 'sharing internationally' is the friendship and links developed between Demelza House in Kent and George Mark House in the USA. In the summer of 1998, a team from the Hospice of Contra Costa in San Francisco visited Demelza House, as they were planning to build the first children's hospice in the USA. So impressed were they with what they saw and the welcome they received that close contact and sharing of ideas followed. The team and architect planning the Californian children's hospice drew on the experience of Demelza House during their consultation and planning process and it was the Chairman of Trustees of Demelza House (who was also the hospice's architect and the

235

father of the young woman who inspired it) who, together with their Company Secretary, dug the first hole for George Mark House at its beautiful site on the outskirts of Oakland. The on-going friendship between Demelza House and George Mark House has led to ideas of exchange visits between the care teams, computer links to enable children in the two hospices to communicate with each other, and even thoughts of exchange visits for families.

Children's hospices come of age

Simplicity is the hallmark of children's hospices. A potential threat to this simplicity and to their ethos could emerge as the hospices move from the pioneering to the mature stage of their development. As they come to occupy an established position within the range of service provision, indeed are seen more as part of mainstream care, we could see what is referred to in the burgeoning literature on palliative care as a process of 'rationalization and routinization' affecting the services, leading to bureaucratization. Informality and flexibility, among the most valued elements of children's hospice care, could be the first victims. A fundamental tenet of hospice care is that services should be adapted to the needs of individuals, not to the convenience of the organization. While individual hospices remain small – and in small intimate settings it is easier to adhere to the basic articles of faith – if their (perhaps extended) services are tied in with larger networks of care, we could see the creation of the sort of rigid systems which are inimical to flexible holistic care.

To take an optimistic stance, however, I would suggest that awareness of a danger is the first step towards circumventing it. It is perfectly possible for children's hospices to provide a vital component of a co-ordinated service of paediatric palliative care without their having to abandon their informing philosophy and defining characteristics. What must be borne in mind at all times is that systems are there to serve, to facilitate the smooth delivery of a service, to protect.

The other side of this coin is the danger that children's hospices could see themselves as somehow exempt from, even above, scrutiny and regulation, as so clearly fired by noble charitable intentions as not to need mundane systems of control and governance. The origins of this, perhaps, lie in the *ad hoc* way in which children's hospices came into being. There is wide recognition nowadays of the important contribution of individual, private endeavour at the local community level in bringing about significant beneficial change. Where such endeavour involves the promulgation of radical new ideas and major fund-raising to build a new service, it is often spearheaded by an exceptional, charismatic individual or small group of energetic Pied Pipers. Their role is indubitably vital in the 'start-up' phase, at the very beginning of a successful venture. This has certainly been the case where children's hospices are concerned. The 'missionary zeal' of the original founders/founding groups generated enthusiastic and vigorous support which often extended far beyond the immediate locality.

Governance and funding

To move smoothly to the mature stage and to secure continued success, however, and to safeguard the aspirations and vision of the original leaders, children's hospices, like any new enterprise, have to ensure that they have in place an appropriate and robust supporting structure and have addressed the problems of succession and governance. This has arguably been less of a problem for the later children's hospices which benefited from the experience of their predecessors and, perhaps, were set up from the outset in a more structured way in terms of management. As in business, the first to enter a 'new market' does not always have the advantage.

In a recent speech on the subject of charities and the government's desire through tax measures to maximize the general public's charitable donations, the Chancellor of the Exchequer made specific mention of hospices and spoke, in this context, of 'civic patriotism'. He thus both recognized the importance of local 'private' initiatives in providing vital services and also acknowledged the praiseworthy financial support given to such initiatives within local communities. The hope is clearly that with additional tax incentives the public will display even greater 'civic patriotism' and give even more generously to their local hospice. It is highly likely that the State will rely ever more heavily on the voluntary sector in the field of hospice care.

All the children's hospices in the UK are registered charities or are incorporated within registered charities. They are thus included within a sector which in England and Wales embraces about 180,000 registered charities with a total annual income approaching £20 billion. Charities have an important role in virtually every area of society and they enjoy important financial privileges (such as tax exemptions and rates relief). In the last two decades, long after the establishment of the welfare state, social and political changes have led to a re-emphasis on the part played by voluntary and charitable organizations.

The last two decades, the period during which children's hospices have been established, have also seen some major changes in the regulatory framework in which charities have to operate. There has been new legislation which has strengthened the position of the Charities Commission for England and Wales, the body responsible for helping charities use their resources effectively and for supervising them to ensure that the public's trust is justified. The most recent of these changes is the introduction of a new Statement of Recommended Practice for Accounting by Charities (SORP) which will define more explicitly the framework within which charities should report on their activities and account for their resources.

'Corporate governance' was a relatively unknown term before the 1990's. It is now highly relevant as the public demands openness, integrity and accountability in all areas of society. Governance of charities – the system by which they are guided, directed and controlled at a strategic level – is an increasingly important issue and presents particular challenges to relatively young organizations, such as children's hospices, which are only now moving from their start-up phase to maturity. The key figures in overseeing the work of charities are their trustees, who are responsible under the law for their general control and administration. Each children's hospice has taken its own approach to the appointment of trustees and the number of trustees varies considerably from one hospice to another; the smallest number is four, the highest eighteen and the average around ten. Typically, the board of trustees of a children's hospice embraces individuals from a wide range of backgrounds who each have some relevant experience or expertise to contribute; these include accountants, lawyers, nurses, special school teachers, retired general practitioners, architects, health authority administrators, paediatricians, physiotherapists, parents and long-term carers. One hospice administrator spoke to me of the importance of keeping a good 'skills mix' on the board of trustees but stressed, too, the importance of having trustees with a genuine interest in the hospice and its work. The director of care at another spoke of the importance of having well-informed and committed trustees; only they, she suggested, are in a position to be 'stewards of the ship' *vis-à-vis* the Charity Commissioners and ambassadors for the hospice in the local community.

Establishing a solid governance structure is important not only to ensure transparency but also to facilitate the development of the organization, the appointment of key staff and management succession. While a project can initially be sustained by the shared ideals of the founders, there comes a time when it is necessary to have more permanent and systematic structures. The challenge then is to ensure that the initial ideals are not stifled by the systems and infrastructure which is needed for proper governance. In this context, it is important to distinguish clearly between the roles of the trustees, who incidentally are unpaid, and those of the team who run the hospice, who need to be given a reasonable degree of freedom in the way in which they manage. The key to maintaining effective governance is regular and open communication between all those involved, a principle which, in my view, needs to be applied throughout the organization.

The costs of running children's hospices are considerable. A survey conducted by the Association of Children's Hospices in 1999 suggests that the average annual cost per bed is approximately £145,000. Bed occupancy rates vary from about 50% to over 90% (although great care needs to be taken in interpreting these crude figures), so that the actual cost of each respite care bed could be regarded as over £200,000 per year for some hospices. It should be stressed, however, that 'costs per bed' cover anything and everything that a hospice provides; in addition to the direct costs associated with caring for children in the hospice, other costs rolled into 'costs per bed' may include home visits, home nursing, bereavement counselling, family support, training, etc. These costs are covered predominantly from charitable donations, and raising money for building, meeting running costs and, in some cases, establishing endowment funds has been a major activity of all children's hospices. Several of them run charity shops and engage in other trading activities. (For this reason, some are constituted as Companies Limited by Guarantee – 'not for profit' companies.) Some hospices receive a degree of statutory support; others, sometimes by choice because they fear that statutory support might come with strings attached and thus compromise their independence, but sometimes simply because none is forthcoming, receive no State funding at all. The average proportion of the funds of a UK children's hospice which comes from the State is at present below 5%.

Current and future issues

It is perhaps not coincidental that, as children's hospices enter the mature stage of their development, children's palliative care should have begun to feature (albeit not yet prominently) in debates on healthcare provision. Interest in palliative care generally has been growing in the years since Helen House opened. Of course, palliative care, though not always explicitly named as such, has always existed, in the sense that there has always been nursing and medical care, with an emphasis on the alleviation of suffering, for the incurably ill. Yet palliative medicine, associated as it has been with 'failure', has traditionally been the poor relation within the field of medicine; it is what 'kicks in' when medical science cannot cure. It could be argued, though, that it is one of the most challenging areas of medicine, where pain and symptom management are tackled in the face of acute awareness of human mortality, and where the importance of the process, as opposed to the outcome (death being inevitable), throws that process into clear relief, requiring the deployment of a wide range of skills beyond the purely medical.

The pioneering work and inspiring example of Dame Cicely Saunders has had a major impact on the status of palliative medicine. It was the success of the hospice movement which she established which led to the concept of hospice care being recognized as a specialty, namely 'palliative medicine', by the Royal College of Physicians (London) in 1987. The founding of the European Association of Palliative Care in 1988 could be seen as an indication of the growing importance attached to the wider area of palliative care. Since its inception the Association has argued for improved professional education and training, for doctors (palliative medicine) but also for nurses, social workers and clergy (palliative care). At a workshop in Brussels in 1993 there was unanimous agreement that strong recommendations should be made to all concerned with medical education that palliative medicine should be included in the syllabus of every medical school.

Thanks in part, I believe, to the emergence of children's hospices and the way that they have, by their very existence, drawn attention to the needs of children with life-limiting illness, palliative care for children is now a recognized, if still under-developed and unco-ordinated, field. Much still remains to be done to establish its position and to guard against patchy provision whereby some children in need of palliative care are victims of the 'postcode lottery'. In this context it is perhaps significant that 50% of health authorities in the UK do not have a palliative care strategy; where they do, it is based largely on the adult model and thus is usually centred around cancer treatment.

Awareness and understanding

One of the greatest and continuing challenges for children's hospices is how best to spread understanding of their work and role and, indeed, how to dispel the misconceptions which still persist. This is vital, not simply for reasons of financial security (to stimulate charitable giving and, possibly, to secure statutory funding) but also to ensure that they reach the children and families they were set up to help.

Initial, but persistent, misunderstanding of what a children's hospice is and, in some quarters, a questioning of their role sometimes verging on hostility, possibly stemmed in part from the success of adult hospices and the widespread understanding of their role, the way in which the concept of hospice care for adults had taken root in the national consciousness. This general understanding of the function of an adult hospice overlay the emerging children's hospices, impeding clear understanding of their rather different role. Adult hospices, many in number and well established by the time Helen House opened, were associated in the public mind with terminal care, usually of cancer patients, the management of pain in the terminal stages of illness, and a high level of medical intervention to control this pain, albeit in a setting more attuned to the broadly spiritual needs of individual patients than a hospital could easily be. At this time, probably the majority of the patients receiving palliative care in an adult hospice would otherwise have been receiving treatment (and/or dying) in hospital. In this sense, the adult hospice was seen as an alternative to hospital.

With this broad understanding of the function of a hospice (and it must be remembered that until 1982 it was not necessary ever to preface the word 'hospice' with the word 'adult'; all hospices were for adults) well rooted in the public consciousness, it is perhaps not surprising that the rather different remit of a children's hospice needed explaining, and continues to need explaining again and again.

It is not that children's hospices 'aren't really dealing with dying people'; rather it is that the nature and time scale of children's life-threatening illness is generally very different from that of adults'. Put crudely, children with a life-limiting condition die more slowly than adults in the terminal stages of cancer. It is for this reason that in a children's hospice there is a much stronger emphasis on respite care and that the imminence of death is not a determining common denominator. Though palliative care may, in a minority of cases, last only a few days or weeks, more commonly it extends over years, with children, often accompanied by members of their family, coming in for short or more extended periods of respite care at regular or irregular intervals, repeatedly over a number of years. These years may see a progressive deterioration in the child's condition, rendering him or her increasingly dependent on parents and carers. The increasing strain, both emotional and physical, that accompanies this deterioration, or simply prolonged uncertainty, makes respite care probably the most important component of the support offered by a children's hospice.

Friendship and support for whole families is a key feature of children's hospice care, more so, I would suggest, than is the case in an adult hospice. There are several reasons for this. The first is the time scale factor mentioned above and the resulting more extended contact with families. The second is that children with a life-limiting illness are usually cared for at home, in a family setting, often with young brothers and sisters; caring sensitively and 'holistically' for a child during his or her stays at the hospice will involve familiarity with the child's normal pattern of care within his or her family setting and understanding of the whole family's expectations, hopes and fears. The third is that many rare life-limiting conditions are 'familial', i.e. there may be more than one affected child within the family.

James and Field,[1] in examining the reasons for the speed with which the adult hospice movement established itself and gained recognition, suggest that its early success depended upon 'a singleness of vision, an intensity of purpose and a narrowness of focus'. These suggested ingredients for successful promulgation of a new idea were, arguably, not lacking when Helen House was set up. However, the mission of the early adult hospices, James and Field go on to suggest, 'resonated with public concern about the care of the dying'. Reflecting on the climate of the time, they speak of 'a public mood of anxiety about death with which the aspirations of the hospices resonated'. They suggest that 'as the ideals and ideas spread, the initial *ad hoc* "separatist" development generated organizational support on a national level which assisted with the dissemination and legitimation of the principles'.

This, for a number of reasons, could not, and cannot, be the case with children's hospices. First, children's hospices address the needs of a comparatively small number of children and families. Whereas the likelihood is that most people will know, or know of, an ill adult who has benefited, or could benefit, from hospice care, or has died in their local

[1] James, N. Field, D. *Social Science and Medicine* 1992; 34(12): 1363–1375.

hospice, this is patently not the case where ill children are concerned. Most children who die after infancy die as the result of an accident or acute illness. Prolonged terminal illness in children is comparatively rare. Though the needs of these children and their families are great, their numbers are relatively small. They are, quite simply, outside most people's experience.

Secondly, the children whom children's hospices seek to help, as well as being relatively few in number, are a largely unseen and unnoticed group. This is because they are in their own homes, cared for by their families, not 'visible statistics' in hospital beds, and not acutely ill and therefore drawing on the acute medical services. Moreover, and importantly, because of the wide range of different and rare life-limiting conditions affecting them, although individually their needs are great, they are not recognized as a discrete group whose needs should be catalogued and met.

Thirdly, children's hospices did not begin in the essentially disruptive (though at the same time obviously hugely creative) way in which the adult ones started. They were not a reaction to, nor a criticism of, an existing service or method of care. Helen House sought to fill a void; it was a response to a clear gap in provision, not a reaction to inadequate or inappropriate provision. For this reason it lacked the controversial element which can serve to spark widespread debate and scrutiny of a new pioneering project and thus usefully highlight its ideals and aims.

These three points all help to explain the comparatively greater difficulty experienced by children's hospices in building understanding of their role and of the need for the service they offer. This is a significant and on-going issue. If the problem is not efficiently and effectively addressed, the losers will be those very children and families that the service was set up to help. Surveys carried out by a number of children's hospices show that the information about hospice services which reaches families usually comes to them via the health, and other, professionals involved in some way with their child's care. It is therefore very important that those professionals should have accurate, detailed and up-to-date information about the services offered by their nearest children's hospice and, ideally, some contact with the hospice. The importance of establishing good links with, and channels of accurate information to, the established providers of medical, social and educational services cannot be overestimated.

In hindsight, the early children's hospices were not all, perhaps, sufficiently active in this area. This is understandable; they were busy establishing their own service; the children and families who came to them had such clear and urgent needs that it was easy to assume that these needs, and how best to address them, must be as obvious to others as they were to those working within the hospice. In the early pioneering days, there was also concern about independence and freedom and how best to safeguard 'hospice ideals'; there was a fear that forging close links with mainstream services would lead to a watering down of the philosophy or even a derailing of aims. Finally – and it must be remembered in this context that children's hospices are largely, and in some cases entirely, funded by voluntary donations – in the early days the hospices were very actively engaged in spreading the word to the general public, on whose generosity their very existence depended. For all these reasons, liaising with the existing statutory services and establishing effective communication was not accorded the priority it perhaps should have been.

The situation today is very different. The need to 'spread the word' in professional circles and to network is widely recognized. Many hospice teams have an individual member with specific responsibility for going out into the field, meeting fellow professionals, establishing links with service providers, arranging visits, and generally disseminating information. Communication is seen as vital if children's hospices are to fulfil their potential within the range of palliative support services for children. The method of communication may vary, not only from hospice to hospice, but also within hospices, according to the circumstances and nature of the communication – most hospices now have 'promotional' videos both for professionals and for families, websites and a wealth of literature – but there is probably no substitute, when establishing fruitful links with professionals, for face-to-face communication.

The difficulty of the educational role facing children's hospices should not be underestimated. When setting up a new and relatively small-scale service (and hospice care for children remains on a small scale, even with the growing number of hospices) it is hard to disseminate information to professionals who are, individually, unlikely to encounter more than one or two potential service users in the entire course of their careers. To take the case of general practitioners, information about hospice care for children will not seem of great relevance alongside, say, information from a drug company about a drug they might prescribe every day.

The human dimension

All children's hospices are small. When Helen House was at the planning stage it was necessary to argue forcefully for small scale and determinedly to look beyond arguments of cost-effectiveness at the construction stage to how best to ensure the hospice's effectiveness in human terms once in operation. Today, the size argument has been convincingly won; size as such is no longer an issue. The experience of the existing children's hospices highlights the importance of small size where holistic care, tailored to individual needs, and the quality of human relationships are at the centre of concerns. Small size quite simply makes it easier to be non-institutional.

The experience of Martin House in Yorkshire (the second children's hospice in the UK) is interesting in this context. When the hospice opened in 1987, it offered respite and/or terminal care to ten children at any one time. However, after five years, the unanimous feeling of the Head Nurse and the care team was that the hospice functioned better, that is to say was able more easily and assuredly to guarantee high-quality care, when it was not operating to full capacity. The decision was taken to reduce the number of children's bedrooms to nine and thereby, at the same time, to create a much-needed small sitting room for families, where a family could withdraw or perhaps have a quiet private conversation with a member of staff or a visiting doctor. Martin House would like further to reduce the number of beds to eight. It is only the demand from families, particularly for respite care, and the feeling of guilt at having more often to turn down a family's request, that has stopped the hospice taking this step.

However, there are other things which militate against the human dimension and against that ethos which is the very characteristic of hospices which families and children most value. Children's hospices have increased awareness of the wide-ranging and complex needs of very ill children and, as they have become established, have been able to spread good practice and disseminate 'hospice principles' into other areas of care throughout the whole field of what is now increasingly often referred to as 'paediatric palliative care'. However, while aspects of the philosophy of hospice care may usefully be translated into, for example, the hospital setting, we perhaps need to beware of a corresponding 'medical backwash' into the hospices.

During the last decade a number of writers on socio-medical issues have highlighted changing trends in the delivery of adult palliative care and suggested that there is a discernible movement towards increasing medicalization of practice. Although, clearly, adult hospices operate differently from children's, inappropriate 'medicalization' of their service is perhaps something that children's hospices need to guard against. The hospices, of course, need to draw on medical expertise, but medical input should have a supportive, not 'directional', function.

Children's hospices rely for medical back-up on the services of local general practitioners. They do not have resident

Medical Directors. Typically, working relationships are established with particular surgeries in the area, whose doctors forge close links with the hospice and, in addition to regular timetabled visits, operate a call-out system. The hospices report favourably on this system, which accords with their home-from-home ethos.

Inevitably, general practitioners who provide these medical services will, over time and through contact with a number of children with rare life-limiting conditions, build up a body of specialist knowledge relating to these conditions, which is often bolstered by dealings with consultants in the field. Thus, they may be in a position to offer or suggest to families medical practices or procedures or new medication which might enhance the quality of their child's life. It would be foolish to suggest that the use of even sophisticated medical practices constitutes *per se* a subversion of the principles of children's hospice care. What is important is the spirit in which such practices are proposed to children and families and the purpose behind their use, if indeed they are used. Communication between the doctor and the child and his or her family is crucial, and it is important that ultimately all decisions rest with the family. A doctor is not abrogating his duty of care by not imposing possibly helpful procedures on a family. Care of a child who, it must be remembered, is normally cared for by his or her family at home, is, and should remain, family-driven.[2] We need to beware of a shift to an 'interventionist approach' with the risk of palliative care practice adopting a disease-centred medical model which might direct the focus away from the fundamental philosophy of holistic care. In sensitive paediatric palliative care, the child remains the focus, not the illness.

Staff development

The members of the care team in a children's hospice are collectively its most valuable resource. Their attitudes and

[2] Worswick, J. *European Journal of Palliative Care* 1994; 2(1): 17–20.

approach set the tone, their responsiveness and sensitivity to the needs, wishes and fears of children and families determine the quality of the care and support these children and families receive. Staff in a children's hospice continue to be selected and employed as much for their personal, as for their professional, skills; in a setting where the quality of human relationships is all-important, professionals cannot claim a monopoly of competence. Having a multidisciplinary, multiskilled team, where equal weight is placed on the diverse skills of different individuals/professionals, serves to break down barriers of authority and status, creating the egalitarian, non-institutional atmosphere which is so valued by families.

Recently, fears have been expressed in relation to adult hospice teams that their multidisciplinary strength could be undermined as a result of the fact that palliative medicine has become a specialty. Doctors or nurses coming into hospice/palliative care and building careers within the specialty, could lose sight of the vision of the multidisciplinary approach in decision-making and leadership, and this multidisciplinary approach, which many believe is crucial to the delivery of holistic care, could be watered down by overly strong medical or nursing direction.

A parallel could perhaps be drawn in the field of children's hospices. As these become an established component of paediatric palliative care provision, there could be a greater expectation among those coming to work within them that professional medical/nursing qualifications will *per se* entitle the holder to seniority within the team, to more say in the direction of the hospice's work. If this misplaced expectation – and by misplaced I mean having no place in the context of holistic hospice care – were allowed to take root and indeed be realized, there could be a change in emphasis in the delivery of children's hospice care. The cohesive strength of the multidisciplinary team could be threatened and the service 'over-professionalized'.

Related to this is an issue which has only come to the fore

as children's hospices have entered the more mature stage of their development. This is the lack of progression, in career terms, for members of the care team within a hospice. Some might argue that this is not really a problem, since those who choose to come and work in a children's hospice are not concerned primarily with career-building. Nevertheless, to address this issue, some children's hospices have introduced, or are considering introducing, special responsibility posts, 'levels' based on length of service, team leader posts, and additional deputy posts. The dilemma, as they see it, is how to preserve the valued team approach while at the same time providing paths of progression for staff.

One approach, perhaps, is to provide personal progression on an individual basis, not on a comparative (and potentially hierarchy-building) basis. This would involve increasing training opportunities for all staff and introducing formal recognition of the multiplicity of skills that individuals develop in the course of their work. A significant number of the valued members of hospice care teams come in without formal qualifications. They and all their colleagues, whatever their background, should have the chance to see the specific skills they acquire and hone in the course of their work 'validated' by formal recognition. If this were widely taken up, qualifications gained would be practice-based, which accords with current trends in medical and nursing training. It is also in line with the expansion of higher education and vocational training generally, the encouragement to study, to update one's skills and pursue life-long learning, and in particular with the increasing certification of skills which accompanies this.

All the members of the care team at Helen House now have the opportunity to work towards the in-house Award in Care. This qualification was introduced in 1997 by the then Head of Care, Mary Thompson, and the member of the team with special responsibility for training, Bronwen Bennett. The comprehensive syllabus for the course was drawn up after widespread discussion during which everyone in the care team had the chance to put forward suggestions as to what should be included. Thus, the 'gestation period' in itself provided an opportunity to think about the whole range of knowledge, skills and competencies involved in paediatric palliative care in a hospice setting, an opportunity which members of the team described as 'very useful' and 'motivating'. The resulting syllabus, incidentally, is an informative reference document for anyone seeking to understand what hospice-based paediatric palliative care entails, and how, indeed, the paediatric model differs from the adult.

The Award in Care course lasts one year. In addition to on-going systematic assessment of their 'hands-on' skills, those taking the course (a maximum of four in any one year) attend a range of lectures and seminars, most of which take place during an intensive training and study fortnight in January when the hospice is closed to children. (Incidentally, these sessions are open to all team members, irrespective of whether they are doing, or plan to do, the Award in Care.) They have evaluation, discussion, and feedback sessions with their mentors and fellow 'students'. They also write a number of reflective essays, choosing the subject of one of these as the topic on which they wish to expand in their extended writing assessment, which goes to the external assessor.

The Award in Care is validated by Oxford Brookes University against the ENB 931, the basic building-block of the Oxford Brookes palliative care course for nurses. This validation, apart from enabling holders of the Award to progress further up the training ladder should they wish to do so, serves to give the Award status beyond Helen House and help outsiders 'situate' the course within palliative care training generally.

The first four Helen House team members to ask to take the Award in Care course all completed it successfully. In October 1998, I was very moved when I was asked to present the first four Awards in our daughter Helen's name, and, to our joy, in her presence.

252

The introduction of the Award in Care is an example of how any perceived lack of progression for those working in hospice-based palliative care can be positively addressed. Individuals work towards formal recognition and certification of the skills and knowledge they have acquired in the workplace, and at the end of the course receive a document that they can take away with them should they ever move on.

Broadening the service
Provision for young adults

Helen House, like the other similar establishments which followed it, was set up and funded as a hospice for children. The early brochures explain to potential users and supporters of the hospice that Helen House welcomes children at any age from birth to sixteen. They go on to state that the hospice is sometimes able to continue to care for children after they have reached sixteen, though it cannot normally take anyone for the first time after that age. Other children's hospices use very similar wording in their literature. The use of words and phrases like 'sometimes' and 'not normally' in relation to care for the slightly older age range, while making it clear that a children's hospice caters primarily for the needs of younger children, also reveals a desire to retain the freedom to be flexible, to consider each case individually. Importantly, the words are also an acknowledgement of the uncertainty surrounding the life-span of children with a life-limiting condition and of the problem of continuing care for such children if and as they move beyond childhood.

On-going support for the older age range has come to the fore in recent years as one of the most sensitive and difficult issues facing children's hospices. What in the early days was recognized as a possibility – namely, that some of the children coming to the hospice for respite would survive beyond childhood – is now an established fact. As time has passed, it has become apparent, too, that some adolescents' conditions seem to stabilize and their life expectancy is therefore increased. What is more, with some life-limiting conditions (for example, cystic fibrosis and some of the childhood cancers) there is now, because of advances in treatment, handling and care, actually significantly increased life expectancy. Since 1981 the average life expectancy for those with cystic fibrosis has risen from sixteen to thirty-one years.

Better nutrition, improved techniques and availability of gastrostomies, advances in the drugs field (more appropriate antibiotics for cystic fibrosis sufferers, more effective anticonvulsant drugs making it possible more easily to control seizures and thereby reduce the risk of repeated further damage to the brain) and the greater availability, within the community, of sophisticated technology which can be highly supportive to children with certain life-limiting conditions – all have contributed to increasing life expectancy. Developments in surgery, too, have played their part, for example, surgery to correct scoliosis in children with muscular dystrophy.

The question facing children's hospices is how far they can realistically cater for the needs of those of their young visitors who live into early adulthood, without running the risk of reducing the support they are able to offer the younger age group, the age group they were originally set up to help. Turning this round, the question is how, in an essentially child-oriented setting, can the needs of young adults be appropriately met? For, just as children are not simply 'mini-adults', as the Association of Children's Hospices is anxious to remind adult hospices seeking to cater for children, no more are young adults simply 'big children'.

It would be hard to imagine anything more difficult than having to tell a young person and his or her family that because of the young person's age, he or she can no longer come for respite to the hospice they have come to regard as home from home. What makes the situation even more difficult is that, however sensitively and gradually any withdrawal of services is handled, and however exhaustive the efforts of hospice staff to help parents explore, over a period of time, other more 'age-appropriate' sources of support, this withdrawal is done in the painful knowledge that there is currently very little suitable respite care available for those moving from paediatric to adult services at nineteen-plus.

It is sensitivity to the needs of this age group, combined with an acute awareness of the current lack of provision to meet these needs, which over recent years has led a number of children's hospices to consider extending their service to include specific, appropriate provision for young adults. The first to establish such provision was Acorns Children's Hospice Trust. At their second children's hospice, which opened in Walsall, Birmingham, in 1999 and has eleven beds, Acorns have a designated area of the building which they call their adolescent unit, which caters exclusively for the fourteen to twenty-five age group. In it there are bedrooms for five young visitors.

In Oxford, Sister Frances announced in 1999 that the Society of All Saints planned to raise money to build a 'respice' for young people between the ages of sixteen and forty, to be called Douglas House. The unit would have seven en suite bedrooms and provide respite care, 'outreach', day care, terminal care and bereavement support. It would be built within the grounds of All Saints Convent.

Martin House in Wetherby, Yorkshire will probably be the first children's hospice to open a specially-designed and completely separate young people's 'wing'. The Martin House trustees have recently approved plans to extend the service the hospice offers; the planned young people's provision will, with the existing children's provision, form 'Martin House, a hospice for children and young people', and the two services will be under the same management and imbued with the same philosophy of care. However, by providing a separate building for them (an adaptation and extension of the Sisters' House in their beautiful grounds, which the Sisters of the Holy Paraclete vacated in 1999) the staff of Martin House are confident that they will be able to provide the sort of environment for the young people they welcome that these young people would themselves choose if free to design their own accommodation. Indeed, in planning the new building, in addition to widespread consultation with architects, planning advisers, service providers, hospice staff and local residents, there has been much discussion with potential young users of the proposed new facility and their families, in a desire to tailor the service closely to their needs.

The new building will have six bedrooms with en suite facilities for young adults in the broadly eighteen to twenty-five age group. All the facilities they will need, including catering, will be under the one roof, though the extensive hospice grounds will be shared by all who come to Martin House, whether children or young adults.

Not all of the existing children's hospices are in a position to build new facilities, or adapt existing ones, to make provision for young adults. Some do not choose to do so, in some instances because they do not feel that this is within their remit (and within their Articles). Moreover, some have reservations about moving into this complex field. However, a growing number seek to cater to some extent for the needs of the older age group, for example, by organizing respite care admissions in such a way as to group similar-age visitors together, scheduling 'teenagers' weekends', 'young people's breaks' and the like.

Family accommodation

When Helen House opened in 1982 it had one small flat with two bedrooms, slightly removed from the heart of the hospice, where parents and relatives could stay. As the years went on, this proved inadequate to accommodate the number of parents and other family members who wished to stay at the hospice to be near their child. In October 1995 Helen House opened a small extension, designed in the same triangular style as the original building and leading off it at the back, to provide additional family accommodation. The extension also contains a large games room to give additional recreational facilities for both children and young people staying at the hospice for respite and their relatives. More recently, in 1998, Helen House bought a terraced house along the road from the hospice which has been refurbished to provide, in addition to office and storage space, yet more family accommodation. This accommodation, comprising two self-contained flats for visiting families, has the advantage of being reassuringly close to the hospice but independent of it. Accommodation and facilities for families has proved to be an important part of the service a children's hospice offers and is an area in which the hospices generally have expanded on the original model.

Sibling support

Related to this practical broadening of the service is what is perhaps best described as a broadening in the field of emotional and psychological support. In the years since Helen House opened, awareness of the needs of the brothers and sisters of life-limited children has grown and deepened. The practical obstacles to their enjoying the full range of activities and experiences that their peers enjoy are many and great. The often complex care needs of their sick brother or sister (or sometimes more than one) impose huge constraints on spontaneous activities, outings, holidays and even entertaining friends, as well as limiting the time parents and children have simply to enjoy each other's company. Moreover, the well brothers and sisters are in a situation which is far removed from the experience of most, if not all, of their friends and peers; this can be very isolating. They are often overwhelmed by feelings of inadequacy, fear, sadness and, possibly, resentment and anger. Yet for most of them, asking for help with their difficulties seems hugely selfish or simply wrong, given the awfulness of their brother or sister's circumstances.

Many children's hospices now have sibling support programmes, set up in an attempt to address the practical and emotional difficulties siblings of very ill children experience. (I use the word 'sibling' as useful shorthand, although I admit to a dislike of the term in the context of hospice care. It would not be readily understood by the young people it is used to describe.) There are increasingly often now members of the care team with special responsibility for sibling support. This support is sometimes on a one-to-one basis, sometimes organized around small groups, and ranges from specially organized activities, outings and, in some cases, short holidays, to the chance simply to talk in relaxed and unhurried circumstances about their fears and feelings. It can be immensely helpful and restorative for well siblings simply to know that their feelings are recognized and acknowledged, that they are 'valid', that they matter. Meeting other young people in broadly similar circumstances and sharing activities with them can alleviate the isolation well siblings often experience. Sometimes friendships develop and siblings from different families choose to keep in touch with each other. The East Anglia Children's Hospice at Milton, Cambridge, has introduced a newsletter, *Chums*, to facilitate this. Bereavement support groups planned specifically with siblings in mind, such as the programme in operation at Martin House, also help siblings feel less alone in times of particular difficulty. Acorns Children's Hospice Trust have recently received a grant from the Diana, Princess of Wales Memorial Fund for a three-year project further to develop the work they have always done with siblings.

Home care

Extending the support they offer within the hospice itself to children and families in their own homes is another way in which some of the children's hospices have sought to broaden their service. Some have always operated in the community; Acorns, Birmingham, for example. (Interestingly, work in the community was originally going to be their core operation.) The service offered by Acorns is not a nursing outreach service; the members of the community team (there are approximately fourteen of them, and they are separate from the in-house care team) are involved mainly in liaising with existing services on behalf of life-limited children and their families, and act as co-ordinators to bring together the help and support families need. It is members of the community team who first visit a family on referral, to establish what their needs are and how best these can be met.

Some hospices, among them Martin House, Hope House in Shropshire, and Helen House, have introduced some measure of home care provision more recently. Some have decided not to enter this field, in some instances for practical reasons. Children's Hospice South West, based at Little Bridge House in North Devon, is an example. The very large area that Children's Hospice South West serves, and the largely rural nature of that area, means that it would be difficult to offer home care to any but the most local of their families. Thus, a two-tier service would develop, which the hospice staff feel would be regrettable. They also prefer to concentrate their resources on care within the hospice and feel that they can be most effective and useful outside the hospice by taking an 'advocacy' role in relation to children and families and encouraging the statutory services to develop home care.

The hospice at Milton, Cambridge believes strongly in working in partnership with other service providers. Though they see home care for the children and families they serve as a priority and have had a small group of dedicated 'outreach co-ordinators' working in this field for the last six years, their approach is that they cannot always deliver the care themselves, but they can try to ensure that it is set up. Effectively, they can seek to 'broker' arrangements on behalf of children and families.

It is important that any children's hospice planning to broaden their service to offer 'hospice care at home' should investigate what is already available in the area they serve and avoid duplicating a service which is operational and viable. They should beware of falling into the way of thinking that they alone must seek to do everything for 'their' families. Exclusivity is rarely productive.

The scheme in operation at Hope House is an interesting model. The home support Hope House offers is very much an addition to the existing in-house service, not a replacement or an adaptation of it; the hospice-based care remains the core activity. Hope House has a community nursing team of four, overseen by the 'community co-ordinator'. This team offers terminal nursing and help in medical emergencies. They might be called in to a family home to help out, for example, when a child is discharged from hospital and there are new, and perhaps daunting, medical procedures for the family and carers to become familiar and confident with, or when a child's condition suddenly deteriorates. Those working for Hope House in the community are very much part of the care team within the hospice (the hospice establishment was increased when home nursing was introduced); this is felt to be important to ensure that the care provided by Hope House is of the same quality and informed by the same guiding principles wherever it is delivered. An interesting idea was to make the community co-ordinator responsible for drawing up all the care team rotas; she is thus in a position to monitor the care experience being acquired by each team member and can, as she sees fit, draw individuals working on the community nursing team back into the hospice to 'top up' their expertise.

Education

Education is another area of development for children's hospices. Sharing with others the expertise and knowledge they have built up working in the field of paediatric palliative care, and themselves learning from those others, is something children's hospices see as important. As the hospices enter their mature phase, there is an increasing emphasis on staff development and training. As they broaden their service, it is important for there to be good communication across the whole range of provision and opportunities for all hospice staff to learn about the work done by others to complement and strengthen what they themselves do. In addition to planning seminars, lectures, study days, open days, workshops and the like, to cater to needs in these different areas, some hospices are now addressing the question of where these educational activities can and should take place, if they are to happen regularly throughout the year. It is important that the privacy of families using the hospice is not compromised.

New hospices can include generous space for meetings, etc. at the planning stage; Ty Hafan, which opened in Cardiff in 1999, has two rooms designed to cater comfortably for meetings and small conferences, within their main complex but accessible from outside the main building. Some established hospices are adapting to meet this need; the hospice at Milton, Cambridge, is currently building an education and training centre with lottery funding, where, in addition to the range of educational activities mentioned above, they plan to run induction courses for new staff and, possibly, arrange talks and discussion groups for families. Demelza House, at Sittingbourne, Kent, recently opened its volunteer centre, again built with the help of lottery funds. The new centre provides facilities, including a large training room, for the staff at Demelza House to train and support hospice volunteers and for visitors to come and learn about the hospice's work, while allowing the children and families to relax within the main body of the house.

Evaluating the service

As well as, perhaps, broadening their service, children's hospices need to ensure that what they are already offering meets families' needs and is in tune with their wishes. They must continue to listen to children and families in order to be responsive, not prescriptive. Getting feedback from families is important in order to guard against complacency. However, many families who bring their child to a hospice have, before then, had relatively little practical help and support in caring for that child; consequently, they are overwhelmed with gratitude for whatever the hospice staff are able to do for them. This, coupled with the fact that the service is free of charge, makes them feel it would be churlish to express any, even slight, dissatisfaction with the support given. This should be borne in mind when eliciting their views and seeking to gauge their satisfaction with the service.

Meaningful feedback is best gathered informally and in an 'on-going' way, in the course of relaxed, unhurried and open-ended conversations between children and families and a member of the care team who knows them well and whom they, for their part, feel at ease with and trust. Grading the hospice service or answering specific questions about it on evaluation forms or questionnaires is daunting for many families, and appropriate questionnaires are, in any case, hard to devise. It is difficult to formulate questions around some of the intangibles that make hospice care what it is, and these intangibles defy the sort of evaluation that forms and questionnaires invite. The danger of seeking always to measure what we value is that we end up only valuing what we can measure.

The way ahead

Children's hospices were highly innovative and came into being as a result of the enterprise, energy and vision of individuals or founding groups. Their roots were to some extent in missionary zeal. A question to be asked as we begin the new millennium is whether an innovative approach can be sustained as time passes and the ventures move further, in time at least, from their origins. Does becoming established, and possibly more integrated into mainstream care, necessarily stifle free thinking and ideals?

I would suggest that it is possible to move *on*, without moving *away*. What is important is that the core function and values remain at the heart of any possibly expanded role. In moving on it is possible to carry the approach and philosophy which informed the foundation of children's hospices into related fields of paediatric care. Becoming established should be seen as providing an opportunity to speak with authority for, and on behalf of, life-limited children and their families. It is to be hoped that children's hospices will seize this opportunity positively to influence, without necessarily seeking themselves to run, other services providing support for the children and families they set out to help.

Index